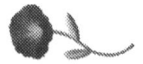

Blessed & Beyond ...

Blessed & Beyond ...

A Passage into Widowhood

JACA DEPRIEST

iUniverse, Inc.

New York Lincoln Shanghai

Blessed & Beyond ...
A Passage into Widowhood

iUniverse books may be ordered through booksellers or by contacting:

iUniverse
2021 Pine Lake Road, Suite 100
Lincoln, NE 68512
www.iuniverse.com
1-800-Authors (1-800-288-4677)

Because of the dynamic nature of the Internet, any Web addresses or links contained in this book may have changed since publication and may no longer be valid.

The views expressed herein are the sole responsibility of the author and do not necessarily reflect the views of iUniverse or its affiliates.

Cover design original artwork by Mary Dana Hardin. Used by permission.
Ms. Hardin's passion for art in began in her mid-teens. Mary Dana works in pen and ink, watercolor and oil. She currently resides in Rock Hill, South Carolina.

ISBN: 978-0-595-41096-5 (pbk)
ISBN: 978-0-595-85455-4 (ebk)

Printed in the United States of America

These words are dedicated to my precious Lawton who awaits me in Heaven. Without the gift of our life together, none of these words would have been possible.

Whether you purchased this book or someone gave it to you, know that God gave this to you, or He gave you a friend who loves you very much. Above all, remember that God, Creator of every living thing, knows the sorrow and pain in your heart. He alone gives comfort and healing, for He alone restores your joy.

Almighty God guides you through difficult times simply and beautifully, even to the end of life and beyond.

It was an incredible time. A time of love. A time of God's grace. A time of God's provision. And a time of great sadness. It's our story told from my perspective and those that surrounded us. I am forever grateful for all of these dear friends and precious family members. The Lord used them in ways I hope I am able to tell you.

This is the story of how Jesus came to take my Lawton home to Heaven.

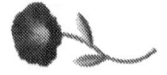

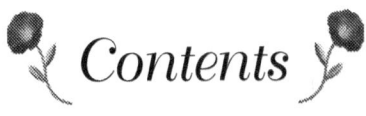

Contents

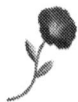

Blessings To

* Debra Ferguson, the first to read my beginning attempt at writing this book. Her inspiration and encouragement for me to continue was unwavering.

* Linda and Jeff Wells who walked by my side every inch of the way. They taught me the true meaning of friendship by their deeds and actions.

* Caran Bevan who is walking her own journey in widowhood. Her ability to present God's perspective has ministered to my heart. Caran is my "voice of reason."

* Lynn Latham who would not take "no" for an answer! Her support, suggestions, and belief that others needed to hear my words were consistently uplifting.

* My niece Cathy who kept asking for more!

* Precious Pat Cameron who is an inspiration to all who know her, especially to me.

* Tricia and Bill Latham who couldn't believe that I would actually stop this labor of love. Their belief in this work has been strong from the beginning.

* All of the Morning Glories, especially the original five—Barbara Adams, Frances Hughes, Evelyn Clites, June Allen, and Barb Saxton. Their precious hearts have ministered to mine in so many ways and have helped develop a ministry for widows.

* Anna Jones who crinkled the pages of the manuscript with her tears as she edited my words. Anna watched and walked with us.

* My co-workers who encourage me every day. They are my family and each is firmly embedded in my heart.

* Donna and Ted Badger who helped put the pieces back together and for making me go beyond what I believed possible.

* Carolyn Jones who joins me in the journey of widowhood bringing a depth of understanding and vision for ministering to and with widows.

* Dr. Manny Zervos—my favorite physician who listened and walked us through. His genuine care and concern for my Lawton's comfort was a forever heart bond—one facing the end of his life and the other beginning a phenomenal God-directed career. Manny is a gifted physician and skilled surgeon who is tireless in his pursuit of a cure for pancreatic cancer.

* My gratitude to those who shared their heart with their words in this book. I am blessed with each of their remembrances of my Lawton.

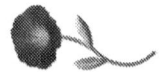

Discovering God's Grace

The Foundation

Over our first twelve years of married life, with its usual bumps in the road and challenges of raising a family, we were happy with our marriage, work, and friends. Before we married, I knew it was a package deal—Lawton and his two children, Lawton "Lawty" Jr. and Fran. We were wed in a little town in Connecticut by a Justice of the Peace. In only a short time, we were settled and involved in Little League, Scouts, and all the other events of raising children, except church.

After five years, Fran moved back with her mother in Alabama. Afterward, we only saw her occasionally. We spent seven years in Connecticut, and then we moved to Florida when the architectural concrete company Lawton worked for closed because of a depressed construction market in the Northeast.

Lawty was involved with his friends, sports, and activities with Scouting. Our life was good as we enjoyed the casual lifestyle offered in Florida. Both of us had jobs that were fulfilling and meaningful. Friends were abundant. Lawton's love of golf developed and deepened as he played several times a week.

In time, I began to wonder if there was something more—more meaningful, more gratifying, more than just the day-to-day "8 to 5" of life. Elusive, there was nothing that I could put my finger on. There was simply an emptiness that I could not identify.

It was then I came to know the Lord in a real and intimate way. I was associated with a group of women who each had a personal relationship with the Lord. These women would tell me how much God loved me, and that He had a plan for my life. They told me how the Lord had given them peace, strength, joy, and fulfillment. Through their encouragement and prayers, I came to have the assurance of eternal life and the assurance I would spend eternity in Heaven with Jesus. This happened by recognizing that we are all sinners, and I personally confessed my sin. With a simple prayer, I asked Jesus to forgive me and to become Lord of my life. At that point, the knowledge that Jesus died for me finally became real. He rose from the grave and ascended to Heaven to be my intercessor with God.

My new friends encouraged me to find a church near my home—a church that taught from the Bible, and taught Jesus is a risen Savior. They encouraged me to find a church that would disciple me and teach that Jesus is very much alive today, living in the hearts of all who trust He is our Redeemer. That was our faithful prayer together. As you might expect, God led me to a church that answered all my needs.

The Building Plan

It was a more than beautiful Easter morning. One of my longtime friends was spending the holiday with us, and she wanted to go to church. I did, too, but since neither she nor I had ever really gone or shown any interest, it was exciting to know that she had the same desire in her heart.

After driving around and checking out several churches in the area and looking at the times of various Easter services, we decided to go to the closest one. It was just around the corner, less than a mile from home. We entered and sat down. Little did I realize that not only would this place become my church, but that these people would become my spiritual family. They were and remain a true reflection of the Body of Christ.

What captured my attention that Easter Sunday was the preacher. With total confidence, he walked to the pulpit, slapped his Bible down and proclaimed, "He's alive. He's alive! Jesus is alive!" His words still resonate in my heart today.

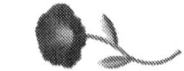

The Building Blocks

Not long after that first visit, a beautiful woman knocked on my door. She introduced herself as being from the church. "Hi, I'm Pat Springer!" We've laughed over the years at that first greeting, which sounded to me so much like Glen Campbell. Our visit was refreshing as she gently guided me in fully understanding and confirming my commitment to the Lord, and I shared how I prayed the simple prayer only weeks earlier.

Not only is Pat a beautiful woman inside and out, but she is gifted in many ways. I remember watching her sing in the choir, her face full of adoration for the Lord as she sang praises and the wonderful old hymns. Pat and her husband, Chuck, became a couple we enjoyed being with, sharing many stories and laughter around the dining table. If you ever wanted a dinner partner, Pat and Chuck were always up to the task. Most Sunday evenings after church would find the four of us at one of the neighborhood restaurants discussing the sermon of the day.

She became my spiritual mother. Sitting under her teaching, leadership and guidance has firmly planted me in His Word and given me a solid understanding of who He is and who He wants to become in me, through me, and for me. So many lives have been touched by her gift of teaching and guidance through His written word. When she prays, you know without a doubt you are at the feet of Jesus. Her life has become a thread through my life, woven by the Lord.

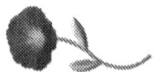

Lawton's Observations

As Lawton watched the change in me as I developed my relationships within the church and the Lord, God began a new work in him. Lawton was one of the multitudes whose life was changed forever by Billy Graham. At nineteen, Lawton worked as an usher at a Billy Graham crusade in St. Louis. It was here he gave his heart to Jesus.

He watched these new people in my life to see if they were genuine, if they truly were who and what they professed to be. As I began making friends in my Sunday school class, they began reaching out to Lawton. Several couples invited us to dinner. Lawton was always asked to the class socials. I remember one Valentine's Day social we were having a bake-off potluck dinner. The husbands were to make desserts that would be judged. It was great fun, and Lawton even won first place with his now-famous red velvet cake. He was a significantly better cook than I have ever been or hoped to be! Lawton even picked up a couple of new golf buddies at some of the gatherings.

So often, I would ask Lawton if he wanted to talk "church." He seldom did. I did, however, manage to get some of my questions out as I sought his wisdom. I wanted to know what it was like to grow up going to church since my family had never attended on a regular basis. I wanted to know what God had done in his life. I asked how you know for sure if you are doing what the Lord wants you to do. I wanted to keep our conversations about God fresh in his mind, because I truly desired to have Lawton next to me at church. I wanted to share worshipping with him. I wanted him to be a part of the church that had so filled my heart with God's love.

Never being one to make hasty decisions (except when shopping), Lawton took almost five years to join this wonderful church and begin serving, learning, and growing. We grew closer together as we grew in the Lord. We developed deep and lasting relationships with the people God brought into our lives.

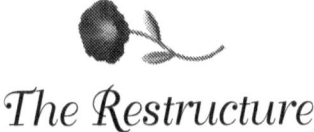

The Restructure

After more than sixteen years with his company, Lawton became another mid-nineties statistic in the downsizing of corporate America. He was a top-notch draftsman both on the board and later on the computer. In some ways, his layoff was an answer to a prayer, but in other ways it was a truly scary time.

I remember asking Lawton if he was excited about what the Lord had in store for him and for us. His reply was, as usual, profound and puzzling.

"Yes and no. I know He's got a plan, but it may not be something I'll like."

God's plan took us on such a journey. Looking back, all I can say is, "Phew!"

For several months after he was laid off, he partnered with a colleague on a contractual basis with offshore work and then for another local company. Interviews took him up and down the East Coast. They were few and far between since his industry was in a weakened condition and no one was hiring. The most viable offer he received was back in Connecticut.

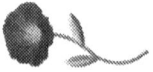

Connecticut–Spring and Summer

It was truly a difficult decision to make. Should he remain here in Brandon working in a part-time capacity for a company with no benefits, or should he pursue the Connecticut option? We prayed, we talked, and we reviewed other possibilities. We discussed the pros and cons of going and not going. Days grew into weeks as we prayed about what to do. God's answer was not clear. Finally, we came to a conclusion. He would go to Connecticut for one year and financially save what we could. Hopefully, after that time, things here would not look so grim, and he'd find work at home. So off to Connecticut he drove.

Hearts already lonely for one another, the feeling was one of being ripped apart. I cried for him all the way to Connecticut.

After he found an apartment, I shipped some household goods and extra furniture to him. He bought a mountain bike and spent the summer riding back and forth to work. Settling in for the year, Lawton toured some of the places we had gone in the early days of our marriage, renewed old friendships, made some new ones, and played a little golf. At best, it was a difficult time. We both missed each other so very much.

It seemed easier for me than for Lawton, because our church family embraced and took care of me during this time. We would see each other only once a month. Either I would go up there, or he would come home on long weekends.

Several months before Lawton's move to the Nutmeg State, on Valentine's Day, our pastor incorporated a renewal of vows into his sermon. It had been my heart's desire to celebrate our twenty-fifth anniversary by renewing our vows, so I started talking to Lawton about it. Along with other couples that day, we stood and renewed our vows. When we sat down, Lawton leaned over to say, "Wouldn't it be funny if we were in Connecticut on our anniversary!"

My response was, "Absolutely not!"

Twenty-five years earlier, we had been married by a Justice of the Peace in Hamden, Connecticut.

Well, as God demonstrated His sense of humor, we celebrated our twenty-fifth wedding anniversary in Connecticut. Our anniversary breakfast was shared with strangers at a railcar diner in Groton, Connecticut. Later that evening, we met one of our longtime friends in a restaurant which had meant so much to us in our early marriage. It was so romantic. You even had to cross through a covered bridge to get to the converted mill on a pond complete with swans and ducks. Little did we know that would be the last night they were open for business. It was perhaps the worst meal we ever had, particularly on such a special occasion as this. Lawton got sick before we even left the building. I was sick the entire next day.

The Cornerstone—"Granny"

After a few months in Connecticut, one of his former colleagues phoned him about an opportunity in North Carolina. He was interested and planned to go for an interview on his next trip home. It would be Labor Day, which was only a week away. The morning of his departure, I received a phone call from one of his sisters, Mary Jane. She told me that their mother, affectionately known to all as Granny, had a stroke and was in the hospital. We decided not to mention her stroke to Lawton until he was back home in Tampa and tell him face to face. News like this is too difficult to share over the phone. She was not doing well and the outlook then was bleak. It was decided that Lawton and Lawty would go to her side. They drove all night to Mobile. Only able to spend two days there, the trip was comforting yet sad to all. Granny had always said that if she was ever sick and Lawton came she knew she would be dying.

Granny, always a fighter, lived six months after her stroke. Mary Jane devotedly cared for her. Lawton's Labor Day visit with Granny would be the last time he would see his mother this side of heaven.

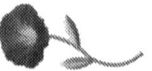

New Foundation in North Carolina

The interview in Raleigh was successful, and Lawton was offered the position. This meant we would be moving, even though I *really* didn't want to leave our home in the Brandon area. I can remember my conversation with the Lord just as clearly as if it was yesterday. I was on the corner of Madison and Tampa Streets in downtown Tampa. I was telling the Lord, one more time, that I truly didn't want to move or to leave everything and start anew. His answer was as clear as a bell.

"Jaca, don't you think that if I choose to move you that I would have gone before you to prepare a place for you? Don't you know that I have it all planned? I'm in North Carolina, too!"

Well, who could argue with that? I fastened my seat belt and held on for the ride. We had no idea at the time, or even during the four years we spent in North Carolina, why the Lord was taking us there. My *Ah-Ha* moment of clarity would only come years later.

We were in Raleigh for seven months while we looked for a home in Oxford. Finally, we found a cute little house to rent, although it was much smaller than we hoped. However, it was in Oxford and close to the office for Lawton. We made our move and started looking for a new church. This was a huge piece of our life we missed so much. Diligently we searched, visiting every church on the map within a twenty mile radius. It took two very long years to find where the Lord wanted us to be. When we found it, the church members embraced us, and we finally felt at home. It was a place where we could worship and grow. The friends we met were extraordinary people. We were able to serve within the body there. I got involved in the budding women's ministry partnering with a precious woman of God named Jackie. She was a gift and a breath of fresh air.

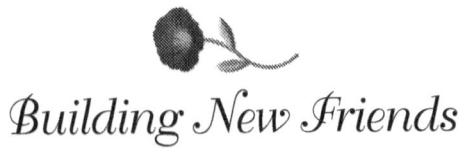

Building New Friends

Jackie's husband, a handsome man named Ed, was attending seminary. He served in the army for many years and answered God's call to full-time ministry. They have two delightful children, Elizabeth and Eddie. Jackie and Ed met in Bible college, and both are extraordinary Bible teachers and speakers.

So many special people came into our lives during the two years we spent at Central Baptist Church. Sherry and Shelly, two pastors' wives, each taught me so much. I never realized how difficult it was to be the wife of a pastor—how vulnerable and alone one can feel. It was a privilege to call them friends.

Shelly was my "secret sister." She always knew when I needed a special touch. There were flowers on my doorstep, cards in the mailbox and surprise gifts in my Sunday school class with my name on them. Shelly was also an incredibly clever woman. She was visiting one afternoon close to Christmas. She asked nonchalantly if I could make fancy bows. "Well, certainly. Do you need one?" I asked. Shelly went out to her car returning with a spool of beautiful ribbon with which I made a fabulous bow. It would be the envy of everyone. A few days later I attended our church's big Christmas dinner, where "secret sisters" would be revealed. In the midst of all of the festive gifts was a huge basket with an incredible bow—my incredible bow. Needless to say, I had to find out who the basket was for. Imagine my surprise when the card said "Jaca!" Shelly and I laughed over that for years.

We met Debra and Eddie at another church we had visited for quite some time. They would become very dear to us. Living in Raleigh for many years they had recently moved back to their hometown of Oxford. They were building a new home on Debra's family farm. One look at Debra and you know she's an extraordinary woman. Her eyes are incredible as she intently listens to your every word. It is evident that she cares about you. Debra is classic, elegant, graceful, and down to earth, always bringing out the best in people. Her thoughtfulness is so genuine. Eddie is warm, friendly, and easygoing. He is a successful entrepreneur and a business visionary. Both Eddie and Debra will be quick to tell you their greatest asset is their two gifted daughters. This family serve the Lord in so many ways and always lend godly support.

Eddie and Lawton even shared in preaching a sermon one Sunday. It was Men's Day at the little country church we attended at the time. Lawton gave his testimony of how he came to receive eternal life. It was the first time I had heard most of the story. He truly enjoyed surprising me and seeing the look on my face. Little did I know how the beginning of my walk with the Lord affected him, and how he watched my relationship with Christ grow. He and Eddie went to Promise Keepers together and spent time on the golf course, and the four of us were in a special Bible study with the Pastor. How extraordinary to be blessed with the precious gift of their friendship.

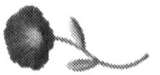

Closer to Jaca's Roots—Virginia

Living in Oxford, we were only three hours from both of my sisters, Fielding and Major, in Virginia. Often we would spend the weekend with them, or they would visit us. We enjoyed holidays together, because we had all been scattered far and wide for most of our married lives. Now it was good to be able to jog up there for a day or two for special times.

Fielding, my older sister, always made sure we did traditional things at holiday time. She'd make sure we served the giblet gravy in Mother's favorite gravy boat or have lobster on her birthday. Major, my other sister, usually looked for something different or spontaneous to do such as touring the "rich and famous" homes in the newly developed Glenmore area of Albemarle County, Virginia. The three of us shared a passion for earrings and loved to find unique pairs for each other.

At one point, my brother-in-law had a significant health issue that hospitalized him for weeks. We would go up almost every weekend to support Fielding and be with the family. So often on the journey home, Lawton and I said that would probably be the last time we would see him alive. We grieved for my sister. Everything she did was for her husband. We didn't think she could go on if he died. Eventually he improved and was given a second chance.

Lawton also had some health problems including a consistently high PSA reading that was discovered during routine blood work which meant potential prostate problems. How fortunate we were to be so close to Duke medical facilities. But still, we felt alone. This was before we found a church and all the support that would have offered. It was just the two of us and the Lord. Oh, how we prayed for his biopsies not to show any cancer. We had some anxious moments, but God in His mercy strengthened and blessed us. There was no evidence of cancer in any of the biopsies over a two year period. Even if there had been, we knew it would be no surprise to God, for He was in control. Electing not to share this experience with Lawty or Fran, we wondered later if this was a wise decision. Don't you want and expect to know when your family is facing a difficult time? Wouldn't you like to pray specifically for them during those times?

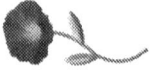

Support Beams—The Puppy Golfers

Lawton's work was good. He had wonderful co-workers, great times on the golf course with them, and they all shared a common love of cigars (that I don't understand). To this day they are still good friends. We called them the "Puppy Golfers" Troy, Andy, Gene, and Sam.

Troy was always available with a kind word. He is a great husband, a fantastic father and ever-smiling. My pet name for him is "T-Roy." Troy is the organizer—the one to get the ball rolling, literally.

Andy, fresh out of college with an engineering degree, was engaged when we first met him. He is tall, handsome and a joy to be around. Andy allowed me to call him Andrew Belew. I chose this name because he would always scratch his back on the doorframe, and it reminded me of the bear in *The Jungle Book*. Today he's a proud father and devoted husband.

Gene is the husband of "Phantom Wife." Whenever we would get together, his wife was usually working, so I started calling her "Phantom Wife." After a year had passed, I finally met her. Now I can't recall her real name. All I remember is "Phantom Wife."

Sam, the quiet one, would join the group whenever he could. Sam is consistent and committed. I'm not sure if his golf game reflects these qualities, but his dedication to his family certainly does. My nickname for him is Steady-on Sam.

These were the core group of Puppy Golfers.

They started the tradition of having golf weekends. The first was early in December 1996. There were about twelve or fourteen of them that went to Myrtle Beach that year. The stories about my Lawton they brought back warmed my heart. He tried so hard to keep up with these youngsters, and for the most part, he really gave them a run for their money. We laughed often at the story Troy told about having to put toilet paper in his ears to block out Lawton's snoring. Lawton had his own room after that first outing. They had a whole new respect for me, too. After the first tournament, it became their tradition to have a spring and a fall weekend. The spring outing took them to Pennsylvania and the fall outing was in Myrtle Beach (better known as "Golf Mecca").

My work was fabulous. I had a wonderful boss who cared so much for his people. It was an interesting position as administrative assistant to the Plant Manager of a well-known textile company. There were many opportunities to minister to co-workers and to form close friendships. Then we received the hard news that our facility would be closing. My heart was breaking. For so many, the work of this plant was a way of life and the only job they ever had. Some had worked there over forty years. With all of these significant changes in our lives, I couldn't help but wonder, "What next?"

Then Lawton told me his former company in Tampa recently called to see if he was interested in returning to work there. I never thought that would have been an option, but once we learned about my job, he began talking to them. Every criterion he proposed was met, and within two months he was back in Tampa. I stayed to sell the house in Oxford, but after three months of separation, it was just too much. We made the decision to leave the house in the hands of our realtor, pack everything, and head south. The house sold within the month.

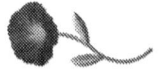

The Network—Florida Revisited

With this sequence of events, it was evident the Lord had a plan, and it was to be executed quickly. Supernaturally things began to fall into place, and here we were back in our house in Brandon (we leased it while we were gone). We were back in our church under great teaching and preaching, and back among our friends. At the time, I didn't know why we were being so blessed, but I was grateful to be home. Only time would reveal the *Ah-Ha* moment—the reason we came home.

I didn't know how the Lord would put the pieces back together, but He did (even better than before we left). It was my plan to return to work after getting resettled in the house in six months or so. The work piece of the puzzle fell into place quickly. The furniture and hundreds of boxes were delivered only two weeks prior when I received a phone call from my friend Debbie. As a staff member of our church, she was in search of a secretary. Well, that certainly was a blessing. Little did I know how huge a blessing it would be as the rest of the story unfolded. It was a whirlwind of a job with not a moment to breathe, but I was learning so much. I was immediately caught up in how God was working in and through the different ministries at the church.

With time passing we quickly regained footing in our home and community. As only the Lord could do, Lawty's position brought him back to Florida. Recently divorced, he could be closer to his children who had returned to Florida some months earlier. With him working so hard opening a new restaurant, we didn't see much of him or the children. Life for most of us was busy and exciting.

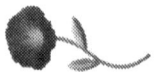

A Stepping Stone—Jaca's Sisters

In late August 2000, while lunching with the girls at work, I received a phone call in the break room. We protected our lunchtime and thought this a real intrusion. It was an emergency call for me. A voice I didn't recognize spoke the words, "My mother just died."

"What?" I asked.

The words came again. "My mother just died."

"Your mother has died? Who is this?" I asked, still not recognizing her voice.

"It's Cathy."

As I tried to process who it was on the other end of the phone, I realized it was my niece Cathy. Then slowly it sunk in. "Fielding is gone?" I asked.

With tears, she said, "Yes."

Everything seemed to be in slow motion as I asked where she was, what had happened, and where her dad was. It was so sudden, so unexpected, and very difficult to understand. As we hung up, I stood there stunned as her words echoed in my head. I remember my co-workers and friends surrounded me and prayed. I called Lawton, and he came home immediately. I called my brother-in-law Bob to comfort him and pray. My Pastor came to my office as I was on the phone with Bob. He gently hugged me and left. He didn't want to intrude as I talked to my family. I couldn't reach my sister Major.

Lawton and I flew to Virginia the next day. It was Labor Day weekend, and everything had to move quickly since she would be laid to rest in the National Cemetery. Two days after Fielding's death, the day she was buried, was Major's sixty-fifth birthday. Fielding's death was unexpected and sudden. She died peacefully in her sleep of an aneurism.

Only a few weeks later, Major discovered a suspicious lump. Examinations and tests followed. By the end of October, she was diagnosed with ovarian cancer. Her journey began. First there was surgery to remove three large tumors followed by chemotherapy. Our family drew together as we had never done before. Lawton and I were able to share how the Lord would carry us through the difficult days of her illness and the grief of Fielding's death. Major handled her illness with grace and great strength. It was my prayer that her strength came from the Lord. I am unsure this was true as I never had the assurance she was a believer.

Like so many others who have chemo, Major began to lose her hair. On our first trip to Virginia to see her after surgery and chemo treatments, she asked if I would finish cutting her hair. So much had fallen out by this time there wasn't much to cut, so we shaved her head. We shed some tears, but we laughed a little. I'll always remember the shape of her head. It was so much like our father's. She always looked like him, but now without her hair it was uncanny. You could definitely tell she was her father's daughter.

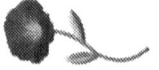

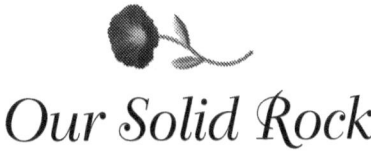

Our Solid Rock

His Illness: The Beginning

In our home and lives, you could see the hand of God at work in all that was said, all that was done, and all that happened. Oh, I pray for these words to tell you and make you feel the presence of the Lord—the bubble of perfect peace that enveloped us. In times of great sadness such as the death of a loved one or grave illness, when your world is shaken to the very core, it is human nature to seek God. I would recall scripture or spend more time in God's Word where I would find His words of comfort and encouragement. I want so much for you to know that peace, that grace, that abundance, that love, that blessing, that time of preparation, and that picture of God's mercy living in us.

For months, my Lawton had not been feeling well. We thought it was stress, as he was unhappy in his work and always kept the goal of retirement in sight. He did all of this for me. You see, he was a good provider.

During these early days, we sought God's answer and tried to cope with the sickness that plagued my Lawton. We knew from blood tests that his iron was low to the point of anemia but had no clue why. His weight loss at first was intentional, then it became rapid and definitely unintentional. In only a few short months, he had lost nearly twenty-five pounds. There were several doctors, lots of advice from well-meaning friends, and many, many prayers for his health.

In July, I felt compelled for Lawton to go to his family reunion, which was held at his Aunt Ruby's home in Missouri. The small voice in my heart kept echoing, "Go to the reunion." Lawton was losing so much weight and was so sick. As we planned the trip, his strength was diminishing so much I felt he needed to go to the hospital. We went to the little community hospital where he was treated for very low potassium. He felt better and we began our journey to the family reunion.

It was a long, difficult trip for him, but somehow I knew it would be important for him to go. Both of his sisters, Mary Jane and Eleanor, would be there. Lots of aunts, uncles, and cousins would be there as well. Aunt Ruby always makes a special effort to keep the family connected. Aunt Ruby's farm is a beautiful spot in Gerald, Missouri not far from St. Louis. We enjoyed the reunion so much. Lawton saw relatives he had not seen in many years.

Our plan was to stay with Aunt Ruby for the better part of a week. After the family reunion, Lawton started getting sick again and was unable to eat or keep anything down. He was absolutely miserable. We decided to begin the trip back to Florida even though he was enjoying the visit with his family.

In what seems now an extraordinarily long time, we finally found a physician that would listen to our situation. We first met with him August 14. He was so thorough in his questions as well as with his methodical procedures for testing.

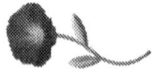

Our September 11, 2001

Four tests were conducted in a very short time frame. On September 11, just as the world was stunned and reeling from the tragedy that struck our nation, we received the diagnosis of a mass on Lawton's pancreas. The doctor did not say the word cancer, but it was evident from the recommendations of doctors. From that moment, our support network kicked in and never left our side. The Lord provided them, He used them, and He gave us a sense of security in Him through them. As they gathered around us to pray, it was evident this was why God moved us back home from North Carolina.

All our doctor would say is that the CT scan that day revealed a mass on the pancreas. He recommended three oncology physicians who would be capable of treating my Lawton. Two I ruled out immediately because of location and experience with Lawton's particular type of cancer.

The next day, I vowed not to leave for work until I had an appointment for Lawton. One of the first things I did was try to contact the doctor at Moffitt Cancer & Research Center in Tampa. Moffitt is a world renowned cancer research center where Lawton was already being monitored for the consistent and continuing elevated PSA readings. My hope was to get a referral from his doctor at Moffitt. Leaving a message for the doctor, I continued searching.

Next on the list was a doctor who was highly regarded at Tampa General Hospital (TGH), Dr. Alexander Rosemurgy. Finally reaching his office, I was able to get an appointment for Lawton the following Monday. Comforted with that, I finally went to work.

Before the end of the day Wednesday, the Moffitt doctor called with his recommendation. He said that Dr. Manny Zervos had agreed to see us on Friday. All I needed to do was call the appointment desk for the time. When I called, much to my surprise, he was in the same practice with Dr. Rosemurgy. We scheduled the Friday appointment instead. "The sooner, the better," I thought.

That evening there was a special Prayer for Our Nation service at church. We went and prayed for those directly impacted by the tragedies only the day before. By then, it was like a very bad dream—not only for us, but also for our country. As we gathered in small groups throughout the Worship Center, the Lord knew exactly who we needed in our little circle of prayer warriors. He sent us Buddy, Jeff, and Linda who were longtime friends and encouragers over the years. Buddy, whose spiritual gift is mercy, serves at our church as Pastor of Hospital and Benevolence. Buddy was one of the first people to reach out to Lawton when we first started attending this church. Buddy worked for the railroad and is an avid race car fan, having worked in that world for a time. Buddy has a name for each of his cars and makes up the cleverest names for most people he works with. For instance, his wife, Judy, is affectionately called "Ha Ha."

Jeff and Linda immediately embraced us, prayed for us and vowed to be by our side through this incredible journey. Linda is the epitome of hospitality. She also sings like a song bird. I love to stand next to her in church hearing her praise the Lord with her beautiful melodic voice. Jeff and Lawton spent many hours on the golf course together. Gentle Jeff is godly, wise, and thoughtful. These are exactly the people you want by your side in a crisis.

My Lawton had a couple of rough days and nights. He would be up and down all night with nausea, pain in his back, and unable to get comfortable. Still he kept working, but he was very tired and weak from battling the ever-present nausea. Finally Friday came, which was the day of our appointment with Dr. Zervos. Lawton was going to work for half a day. It was stormy outside and a predicted hurricane was approaching. Dr. Zervos' office called and cancelled the appointment due to the severe weather. We were devastated. Could we keep the Monday appointment? They weren't sure. I'd have to call on Monday to confirm that.

Not thirty minutes later, the phone rang. It was Dr. Zervos calling to apologize for the cancellation. After telling him how sick my Lawton was and describing how difficult the previous days and weeks had been, he said the only way he could see him that day was to bring him to TGH Emergency Room. He would meet us there. That was the beginning of a six-month journey that would reveal God's absolute love, incredible mercy, and abounding grace. It would be a journey that brought us closer to our family than we ever thought—a journey that would bind our hearts together as never before.

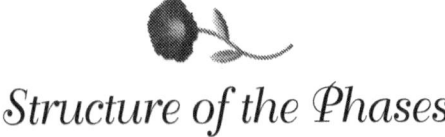

Structure of the Phases

Two of our biggest supporters and extraordinary prayer warriors took us to the hospital. They were Debbie, a woman of God, and Joy, our very own R.N., medical translator, and guide. It was a stormy day even though the predicted hurricane was downgraded to a tropical storm. During the ride to the hospital, it seemed prophetic. We listened to Dr. Billy Graham's radio broadcast of the National Prayer for Our Nation Service in Washington DC. It was September 14 (exactly one month since we met with the first doctor). The words Dr. Graham spoke seemed like they were directed specifically to Lawton and me, not the entire nation. His words, as they always seem to do, brought great comfort and assurance that the Lord was still in control both globally and personally, and that He was and is a personal God.

We registered in the ER and awaited Dr. Zervos. Thinking I'd roam the halls of the hospital, hoping to find our doctor and praying he'd come quickly, I began to pace and wander. I passed a young doctor all crisp and starched in his pure white doctor coat. The University of South Florida Medical emblem on his coat seemed to be blinking and catching my eye. Then I saw his name—Dr. Emmanuel Zervos. His very name was comfort—Emmanuel. God was with us offering assurance. During the days, weeks, and months to come, he and my Lawton formed a strong bond. He soon became our Manny.

So much happened that day including a fourteen-hour visit in the ER. Manny thought Lawton looked too good to be so sick and wasn't sure he could admit and treat him. Blood work revealed that Lawton's potassium was once again extremely low due to dehydration. We were admitted to the ER. Manny reviewed all of the records we brought with us. His recommendation was to utilize a new piece of X-ray equipment that would give a 3-D image of the pancreas for a more definite diagnosis. After several failed attempts, because the equipment was not functioning properly, it was decided that Lawton would have to come back another time for this procedure.

Early in our ER stay, the phone rang in our little cubicle. It was one of our favorite people. I have always called him our other son—Kirk. How he loved my precious Lawton. He was and still is a very dear part of our family and a major part of our lives. What a surprise to hear his voice. Lawty had called him to check on us. Knowing we were going to be there for quite a while, we invited him to join us if he had nothing better to do on that stormy day. Kirk hadn't seen "Mr. D." in some time and was shocked at his appearance because of all the weight loss. It was through Kirk that Lawty finally realized his dad was truly sick, and he needed to pay closer attention to him.

We saw all kinds of things in the ER that day. Debbie thought it was nothing like TV. The nurses told her to just wait. You have to know Debbie to appreciate the fact that she was even there at all—she just doesn't "do" hospitals. That would definitely change.

I remember well one of the conversations of the evening. It was just the three of us—Joy, Dr. Zervos, and me. She asked Dr. Zervos how much time we were looking at for my Lawton. His response was sobering. He said he was not certain, but if he had to say, it would probably be around six months. It took our breath away but not our hope. We made him aware we wanted to know everything, and we did not want him to hold anything back. What he knew, we wanted to know. We cried. We prayed.

About midnight, Debbie and Joy went home. Joy's husband came to pick them up, and she left her SUV so we could get home once Lawton was discharged. Fourteen hours after our arrival at Tampa General he was stable enough to go home. It was the wee hours of the morning, and we were exhausted.

We are troubled on every side, yet not distressed; we are per-
plexed, but not in despair
Persecuted, but not forsaken; cast down, but not destroyed. (2
Cor. 4:8–9)

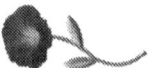

Family First—Lawton's Daughter

Over the years, we did not have a particularly good relationship with
Fran. It was always on again, off again, but it was mostly off. We
always prayed for her and her family, but for reasons only Fran
knows, she withheld her relationship with her father. Often Lawton
and I would talk about when and how she might come back into our
life. Now, she was back. With the diagnosis of his illness came a
phone call from her. I was so pleased she called, but I made it clear in
a very definite manner this was not the time for a high maintenance
relationship. Furthermore, I would be fiercely protective concerning
his healthcare. If there came a time I felt their relationship was anything other than nurturing and loving, she would not be welcome in
our home. I knew that sounded harsh, but it needed to be said. She
accepted my words with the promise her intentions were only to talk
to her dad and see where it went from there.

We invited her to come anytime, and she did. She came immediately. You could see the concern in her eyes, even fear, at the possibility of losing her father. Even though she wasn't part of our lives, she
always knew her daddy was there if she needed him. Now with his illness, that assurance was being taken away. The visit was bathed in
much prayer. Her visit was so very sweet.

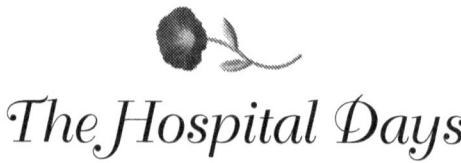

The Hospital Days

The next days were a little better because of the potassium Lawton received, much like the treatment he received in July. But in only a few days the nausea returned, he had no appetite, and he was fatigued and weak. By Tuesday I was begging the doctors to admit Lawton to the hospital primarily for the 3-D X-ray and a better diagnosis. Finally they agreed. We were escorted to TGH by Linda and Jeff and met in the admitting lobby by Buddy and Pat Springer. As we were guided through the admission process, those four stayed throughout the day.

We had to wait for a room as there was an emergency in process on the floor where we were assigned. We occupied ourselves by admiring the view of Tampa Bay from the eighth floor of Tampa General. Jeff and Buddy would see updates about our room from the nurses while Linda and Pat talked to us about our days leading up to our very personal 9/11. Mostly we just sat and waited for our room to be available. All of us realized how serious Lawton's condition was. We didn't need conversation. Just being with one another was a great comfort. I knew each individual heart was having a conversation with the Lord. As the day drew on, Jeff and Linda remained with us, keeping me fed, encouraged, and focused. They prayed with us and even cried a bit with us. It would be a long journey for them as well.

There was not much to do on that first day, September 18. IVs started to replace Lawton's fluids. He also had blood work, medical history, and a visit with the doctors. That day during rounds, a plan of treatment was outlined.

I didn't really keep a journal; however, as I was waiting for Lawton to have an X-ray and CT scan late on September 20, 2001, I realized this was indeed going to be a very long and intense journey. These are some of my notes as I reflected on the days past:

> *It has been nine days since the terrorist attack on America and nine days since our diagnosis of the mass on Lawton's pancreas. After the endoscopy, colonoscopy, X-ray of his intestines, the final test, and a CT scan revealed the mass on his pancreas.*
>
> *The events from Tuesday, September 18, 2001, have changed our lives forever. Joy and Debbie came late in the evening. While we were in X-ray getting the much awaited 3-D CT scan, Kirk arrived with dinner for me. His thoughtfulness always blessed us.*
>
> *Our nurse for the night was Erica. She made our first night at Tampa General most comfortable.*

I knew that Erica was a special nurse when she was tucking Lawton in on our first night, because she said she almost joined the group praying over Lawton that evening. Her warm and friendly smile was genuine. She laughed easily and quickly made us feel comfortable in a strange environment. As a single mom, Erica was continuing her education to earn her RN. She was skilled and confident in caring for her patients. We were blessed to be beneficiaries of her training.

Erica and I had dinner recently, and she shared with me conversations she'd had with my Lawton. "He was always concerned about you," she told me. "He wanted you not to be sad but to draw strength from God. He was not afraid of what lay ahead for him. Lawton just wanted to make sure you were going to be okay."

The next day, Wednesday, our friend Mary Etta arrived about 9:30 AM bearing fresh clothes for me and a wonderful breakfast. We anxiously awaited the biopsy. Dr. Zervos stopped by and told us he would check on the CT film and come back after studying it. Beautiful flowers from the precious support staff at work arrived about fifteen minutes before Dr. Zervos returned.

When Manny returned, he indicated that he wished to speak with us privately as our friend Mary Etta was in the room with us. We didn't feel it necessary for her to leave as extra ears are always helpful. Manny sat in a chair opposite Lawton and me as we sat on the edge of the bed. He had to look up slightly to us to have eye contact. His news was devastating. With Mary Etta by our side, he explained the situation.

Manny told us that it was very serious. The biopsy was atypical. In other words, inconclusive, not showing that it was benign or cancerous. It was as if we were moving through Jell-o. Slowly the Jell-o was liquefying and we could breathe a little. Manny continued to present words in a different way so we were able to hear with clarity and understanding. On his third attempt, with tears beginning to appear in his own eyes, his words were crystal clear, and we began to understand what we were facing. It finally clicked; we came out of the Jell-o into the real world. Mary Etta, on the other hand, understood immediately. Tears were streaming down her face.

He told us that my Lawton had either glandular cancer or a neuroendocrine tumor, neither of which was operable. Not only was his pancreatic tumor wrapped around a blood vessel at the head of his pancreas, but there were spots on his liver as well. If the tumor was neuroendocrine, then the treatment protocol would be chemotherapy. If the tumor was glandular, chemotherapy would extend his life perhaps six weeks. The last option was to make Lawton as comfortable as possible, maintain quality of life, and work on getting his affairs in order.

Through the tears and heavy hearts, we found peace that only the Lord can provide. With misty eyes, Dr. Zervos explained what the next steps would be. Mary Etta prayed with us while we processed the news. Lawton's faith was unshaken. I, on the other hand, was in shock.

Someone, perhaps Mary Etta, called our church family, and they quickly rallied to be at our side with many prayers, hugs, and words of encouragement. Lawty was here in a matter of two hours, normally close to a three-hour drive. Other family called, and again there were tears and prayers. That Wednesday's events are mostly a blur except for the words Lawton had for his son during some quiet time together. He said, "Even though the news is not good, and it probably means there isn't much time left, we have been given an incredible gift—time to talk and say things that need to be said, time to make memories, and yes, to say good-bye. We have time—unlike the people who were killed in the attack on America."

Lawton's sister Mary Jane was scheduled to come from Mobile for our church women's retreat. She came to be by his side, staying just over three weeks. She wanted to stay longer but decided she needed to go home and drive back a few weeks later. Mary Jane had made it perfectly clear that she would be by our side as long as we needed her. What a blessing her companionship would be in the days, weeks, and months to come.

Unsung Heroines

There are so many stories from our numerous hospitalizations. Putting each one in sequential order is nearly impossible as they happened so fast and on a daily basis. One of those stories is about the special nurses from the TGH Angiogram area. We were there often checking on drains, liver biopsies, and procedures too numerous to list. The first time we were there was to have the needle biopsy of the liver which would give us a definite diagnosis. Treatment could not proceed until this information was obtained. Lawton had to be awake throughout the process because of the nature of the biopsy and the position of the tumor in relation to the liver.

Buddy was there from the church as well as others. As they were wheeling Lawton into X-ray, we stopped them in order to pray. From that moment, God was absolutely welcome in that place. You could *see* a difference in the nurses. Oh how I wish I could remember their names! I'll never forget their faces or their hearts.

One day we were awaiting our turn which meant waiting all day to be seen for another angiogram. The hospital transport team never came to get us. Our floor nurses were probably really tired of us asking when we were scheduled for the procedure. Naturally, Lawton had to fast for the procedure. It was not a very good day for any of us, especially my Lawton.

Shortly after 5:00 PM two precious nurses from Angio came to our room to apologize for not getting us in during the day. They explained that there were emergencies and other scheduled patients took longer than planned. They promised we would be the first patient seen the following day. They did not need to take the time to come to us. It was the Lord's way of verifying He indeed was still in control, loving, merciful, and kind. He used these wonderful women to share His love. I will always praise Him for the people He brought into our lives during our time in that magnificent hospital.

Lawton was discharged from TGH on September 25, just in time for his birthday.

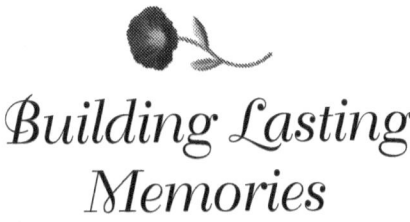

Building Lasting Memories

The Last Birthday Party

Linda, one of my dearest friends, and I talked. She felt every bit of every emotion that my Lawton and I felt during this time. She designed my Lawton's last birthday. They searched far and wide for just the right birthday cake—an ice-cream cake with vanilla ice cream and white cake. Lawton's appetite was so diminished, but he would and could eat ice cream. It was one of our all time favorites, and he was a vanilla guy.

Linda planned it down to the special birthday napkins and candles. We surprised our Lawton, but one of the biggest surprises was Lawty popping in (after the three hour drive) to be with his dad for a few minutes on his sixty-fourth birthday. He couldn't stay long since he had to work later in the afternoon. So there we were at 10:00 in the morning, having a big birthday celebration with Mary Jane, Lawty, Linda, Jeff, me, and my Lawton. We all knew it was his last birthday and wanted to make this a very special day for him and a precious memory for us.

Throughout the day, folks dropped by for a hug and special greeting. A gang of women from my office stopped by to sing. It was a delightful day.

Since Fran and her son Nicholas were coming on the weekend, we saved some of the birthday cake so they could share a belated birthday celebration. I set aside one slice for me. I kept it in the freezer for a very special occasion.

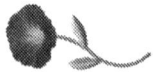

Revolving Doors in October and November

We had a follow-up visit with Dr. Zervos on Monday, October 1. We learned the biopsy came back atypical, which simply meant no clear diagnosis could be made. Manny offered a couple of options. Since eating was difficult for Lawton, we could either have a feeding tube inserted, or he could do a stomach bypass procedure (a jejunostomy). Having this particular surgery would enable Manny to get a clear biopsy as well as enhance Lawton's quality of life by being able to eat normally. He had the surgery on the following Wednesday.

Before he was discharged a week later, he received a med port is a device placed surgically under the skin to avoid multiple IVs in order to facilitate chemo treatments. Lawton met the criteria, so we accepted the opportunity to participate in a study for pancreatic cancer. Lawton believed his participation in the study might benefit someone in the future.

My sister Major came for a visit the day after my Lawton came home from the jejunostomy. It was great having sisters to pamper and spoil my Lawton after all that he had been through in the last month. Mary Jane did lots of cooking; Major did lots of massaging of Lawton's feet, neck, and back. She also arranged and rearranged the multitude of flowers we received over the last several weeks. Our home looked like an upscale florist shop. We had several after-midnight cups of hot chocolate together. Both Major and Mary Jane had experienced cancer and now so was my Lawton. I was the only oddball in the bunch.

Lawty would call every day when he was unable to come over. His work kept him busy and hours were irregular. Shortly after Lawton's birthday, several days passed when we didn't hear from Lawty. It was highly unusual not having a phone call, a visit, or anything. When he finally called, the news was devastating. He and his wife had separated. We knew that he was having serious problems in his new marriage. He was in a situation where he could not call us and didn't want his unfortunate circumstance to burden us now.

For the months that followed, things were as bad as they could get. He was unable to even go into his own home, having to make other living arrangements.

We couldn't dwell on it; only the Lord could heal. Our role was to encourage and support Lawty through this unbelievably difficult time, totally relying on Jehovah Jireh, our provider.

> Come to Me, all who are weary and heavy-laden, and I will give you rest. (Matt. 11:28)

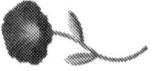

The Missionaries

Our church was having its third annual Global Impact Celebration, a missionary conference. Dozens of missionaries from all over the world come to participate in our mission's emphasis. Each year is spectacular, but this year was extra special.

A family we came to know and love while in North Carolina was invited to be one of the guest missionaries. They had been serving in Kenya for two years on their first assignment. We loved being with them and experiencing world missions up close and personal.

The special worship services, time spent with the missionary families, and unique outings such as the dinner cruise one tropical and balmy night were absolutely perfect. This was the last time Lawton was well enough to go to church. How he found the strength and energy to do all that he did was an encouragement to those around us.

On October 22, we went back to TGH to have a kidney stone removed that was discovered in September by Dr. Seinge after a routine visit. We were only in the hospital overnight.

Seven days later was Lawton's first visit with the oncologist, and we scheduled the first chemo treatment for November 5. He was having problems with his digestion, and it was recommended he get a bile stint to facilitate drainage. I remember asking Dr. Zervos what the next big hurdle would be in the big picture of his illness. He said it would be infection. The symptoms would be fever, jaundice, and nausea.

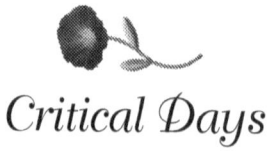

Critical Days

Lawton's sister Eleanor arrived from Massachusetts on November 8. We picked her up at the Tampa International Airport, stopping for dinner on the way home. Mary Jane, his other sister, returned to be there during Eleanor's visit. It was a good thing because we were about to face a major life-threatening aspect of Lawton's illness. All that day Lawton was feeling lousy with pain and nausea. When we got home from dinner, I checked his temperature. It was 102°. Calling our doctor immediately, he told us to come in right away for a direct admission.

As we got to our hospital room that night, Lawton began having unbelievable chills, shaking uncontrollably, and feeling miserable. I prayed with him asking God to make him comfortable and to keep him warm. As the night progressed, I watched the fog roll in from

Tampa Bay, blurring the downtown Tampa skyline. Actually, I couldn't tell if it was the fog blurring the scene before me or if it was my tears. The words Dr. Zervos had spoken only days before echoed in my ears. "Infection will be the next threat and hurdle."

For the next three weeks we battled an infection. Dr. Zervos gently made it clear to us this was a life-threatening situation. He treated Lawton with the most potent antibiotics available. Lawton had severe jaundice and increased chills that caused him to shake uncontrollably. Eventually he was able to tell when they would start so we could call for morphine which would lessen the severity and duration of the episode.

Mary Jane and I had a routine. We would kick into action when the chills began. Very much against protocol and hospital regulations, we heated blankets in the microwave and put them next to Lawton's now tiny body, piled pillows around him to keep the heat in, and added blanket upon blanket. It worked and made him just a little more comfortable or at least able to tolerate the chills while they lasted. Many times he would have ten or twelve blankets piled on him. He looked like "marshmallow man" with a little orange face. Because of the jaundice, I nicknamed him "Sweet Potato Man." He had lost too much weight to be called "Pumpkin Man."

Once when he was having a chill spell, we had guests. They sat there in awe as Mary Jane and I launched into our routine. Thirty minutes later, they asked if this happened often. "Yep," we said.

Their only comment was, "Impressive!"

We were there so long this time all the nurses knew when I came to the door, I needed something immediately. They were always quick to serve and respond. I think we had each nurse working on that floor at least once during all of our hospitalizations. Lawty, Fran, and their children would come as often as they could, usually on weekends.

Our favorite view from the hospital room was of downtown Tampa. Most people preferred the Bay side, but not us. We looked forward to sunset and the lights appearing slowly, one by one. Watching throughout the long nights, we enjoyed the lights, the mist, the twinkle through the rain, and the peaceful calm that came over the city.

Whenever you think of your hometown, do you remember the terrain, the "Welcome To ..." sign, the skyline or other special characteristic of your home? For me, it's the gentle beauty of the Tampa skyline. I would look for it as my flight approached or as I drove into town seeing the first glimpse as I reached the top of the bridge or around the curve on the expressway. The old and new blended beautifully. The University of Tampa would gleam with its golden minarets. There's the Italian marble of the second tallest building or the gently sloping green roof of the tallest building. There is one building with unique pyramid lights at the top. On the Fourth of July, it's red, white, and blue, and on Christmas the lights alternate between the green and white of a Christmas tree or the red and white of Santa's hat.

One night we realized the lights were out and were concerned being so close to 9/11. The next night we anxiously waited for the lights to appear. And appear they did. Watching off and on all evening, we saw the lights went out sometime after 11:00 PM. We wanted to know the exact time and if it was consistent. Then it became a game—what time did they actually go out? It's incredibly difficult to get a good night's sleep in the hospital. But, it's even more difficult to stay awake when you particularly want to see something and are waiting and watching for it. Sometimes I would stay awake, sometimes it was Mary Jane, but mostly it was my Lawton. Distractions are good sometimes, I guess.

Our window also overlooked the helicopter pad. Often the stillness of the night was interrupted by the *thwap-thwap-thwap* of the chopper lifting off to a late-night rescue. During the day, before we heard the sound of the helicopter blades, we would see the birds abruptly taking flight and soaring. It was a sure indication of either an incoming chopper or revving engines preparing for takeoff. You know the grandchildren enjoyed the excitement of seeing those arrivals and departures. There wasn't much to occupy them during the hospital visits with Grandpa.

During one of our hospital stays, there was a lunar eclipse at 3:00 AM. My Lawton was determined to see the eclipse. We went traipsing down the hospital corridors trying to find a dark enough room without any patients so we would have a good view of the celestial event. The nurses thought we were nut cases until they knew what we were doing. Well, we never did get to see the eclipse. With the bright lights inside and outside of the hospital it was impossible to see anything but your reflection in the window.

Thanksgiving and the Hall Pass

Our heart's desire was to be home for Thanksgiving. We had hoped Lawton would be strong and well enough to be discharged. There was still some concern since he had received several blood transfusions. It is protocol to keep a patient for a designated time after receiving a blood transfusion. We knew he could be discharged soon. We really wanted to be home since all of the family was coming. Lawty and Fran planned dinner, and all we needed to do was be there. If we were not out of the hospital by Thanksgiving, they would bring Thanksgiving to us. We begged Manny to give us at least a hall pass for the afternoon. Reluctantly he did. He hesitated because Lawton received two units of blood the day before, and he needed to be under his care for another twenty-four hours.

We disconnected the medical equipment, got a wheelchair and a nurse to bring him down to the car, and headed for home. It was a magnificent feast and a blessing to be home, even briefly. Having our family around us, loving one another through this difficult time was something we were so very thankful for. We took lots of pictures of everybody. In his hospital gown, my Lawton looked so happy with grandchildren hugging, kissing, and crawling all over him.

On the way back to the hospital, Lawton was chilled to the bone. He wanted me to turn up the heat in the car. "Turn it up more … that's not enough … I'm still cold." We wrapped him in a blanket. "Won't that heater crank up any higher?" he wanted to know. It was over 95° in the car. Mary Jane and I, both prone to significant hot flashes, were not enjoying the sauna. But it wasn't about us.

Home Sweet Home

The very next day, Manny thought Lawton was stable enough to be discharged with home healthcare. We were thrilled to finally be going home. Finally, time to be together alone, no daily blood tests at 4:00 AM, food that was home cooked and hot. We had missed our own bed, being able to snuggle, go outside in the sunshine, play with the dog. Rest.

However, it turned out to be a nightmare. Either our expectations of home healthcare were too high or the skill of the nurses with this organization was insufficient for our needs. Somehow communication from the hospital was not received by the home health provider. There was such confusion with the healthcare nurse, the pharmaceuticals, and everything. They were not prepared to handle a simple biliary drain tube from his stomach or even to provide supplies for it. The antibiotic he needed would not even be delivered until late the following day.

The whole situation was so upsetting to Lawton he asked to be taken back to the hospital until it could be straightened out. So back we went for almost another week. After once again getting him stabilized, we came home with another home healthcare company. This one proved not much better. All the nurse talked about was how long our insurance would pay for her to come, and after that I was on my own. We quickly made arrangements for Manny to write a prescription for Hospice and called them to begin providing his care on December 5.

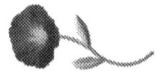

Keeping it Together–Hospice ...

From the first time a Hospice representative entered our home, I knew beyond a shadow of a doubt this was a very special organization with incredible people to care for my Lawton. Once all of the paperwork was complete, a nurse was scheduled to come the next day, evaluate Lawton, and spend time getting to know us.

She was so very caring and thoughtful. Her name was Linda. It was evident from the beginning she loved the Lord and served him through her work and life. In the days ahead, we became very close. On her days off we missed her, but the others who came in her place were wonderful as well. Each one would care for Lawton and then spend time with me answering my many questions, comforting me, quieting my fears, and showing me how to change his IVs, dressings, give medications and injections.

A counselor spent time with us too. Her services were available to us and any family member twenty-four/seven. We had concerns with one of our grandsons, and she made a special Sunday visit just for him when he was in town. It was a great comfort to him. I know he had many questions. He listened to stories she told about other children in similar family situations and the experiences she had. She helped all of us process the fact that Lawton was dying.

I can honestly say each Hospice representative that came into our home had a vibrant, personal relationship with the Lord. This was most comforting to all of us.

If I had to pick one thing Hospice provided it would be peace of mind that no matter the time of day, if we needed assistance, they were available either by phone or home visit. One time at 3:00 AM when I thought I broke or compromised his IV-PIC line, and I could not focus on their directions over the phone, a nurse was on our doorstep within the hour.

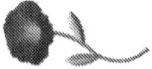

The Last Visits—Saying Good-Bye

The Christmas Stories

About a week after we were with Hospice, I received a phone call from a precious sister in Christ from work. Eloise (whom I affectionately call "Elo-weegie") asked if a couple of people from the office could stop by the next day to check up on "us kids." She said they would be there at noon. Of course they could come, and if it was not a good day for Lawton, I'd let them know to select another day. It was a Tuesday; Mary Jane went home the day before to be with her family for Christmas. It was the two of us, and I was really nervous about taking care of my Lawton all by myself. We started the day with our usual breakfast and changing of the IVs, medications, and all other medically related items that would become routine in the days ahead. Since company was expected, we made sure Lawton was all shiny, polished, showered, shaved, and his most presentable handsome self.

Promptly at noon the doorbell rang. When I opened the door I was greeted with almost the complete staff of our church. They came to sing Christmas carols. We managed to get Lawton to the door, IV pole and all. Remembering this I still have tears in my eyes and a heart full of love for these people. Just imagine, in the midst of the saddest time of your life, and in your front yard is the Body of Christ singing praises to the Lord, bringing hope, love, and a much-needed hug. They sang for about twenty minutes. We stood there and wept, softly saying to each other, "How precious of them to do this."

We were absolutely blown away with the tenderness on each face. After the singing, they came one by one to give us a big hug and whisper something encouraging and loving in our ears. I don't know how I had the presence of mind to capture this moment on film, but the picture says it all.

This was a magnificent gift to us. For the remainder of his days, my Lawton kept saying, "I can't believe they did that … why did they do that … how did they do that … what a wonderful thing for them to do!"

I have the picture in my office. When people notice or comment on it, I share this story, and those who hear the story always have tears in their eyes. Even our neighbors still talk about when the "church people" came to sing Christmas carols to us.

Again, this was proof the Lord's mercies are new every day. He gives us what we need when we need it. On that Tuesday, we needed a portrait of the Body of Christ and to know we weren't alone.

> This I recall to my mind, therefore, I have hope
> The Lord's loving kindnesses indeed never cease, for His compassions never fail.
> They are new every morning; Great is Thy faithfulness.
> "The Lord is my portion," says my soul: "Therefore I have hope in Him."
> The Lord is good to those who wait for Him, to the person who seeks Him. (Lam. 3:21–25)

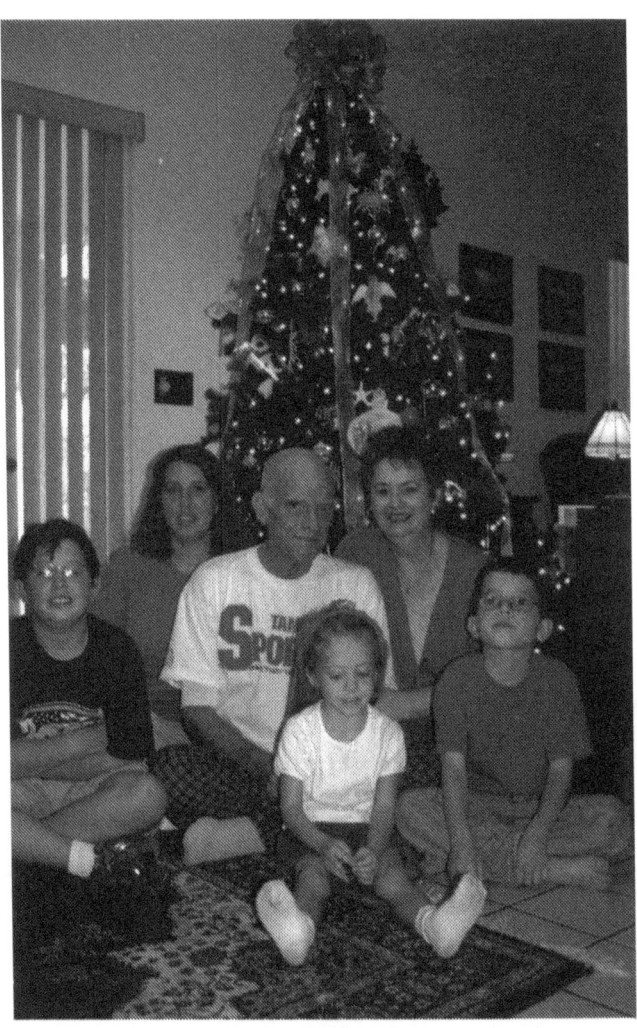

Our last Christmas together.
Lawton, Jaca, Fran, Nicholas, Jennings, and Kendall

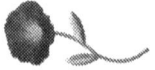

The Christmas Tree

Knowing this was the last Christmas for all of us together, it was so important to put up our tree. I didn't want it in the living room where we always put it. The tree needed to be in the family room where we lived. Fran and Nicholas decorated the tree.

As with all families, it seems there are stories associated with each ornament. We are no different. Nicholas, who was soon to be twelve, had not spent a Christmas with his grandfather for years and years. He took great delight in examining each ornament, listening to the story, and with great care putting it on the tree. It was an incredible Christmas for all of us. Our prayer was for my Lawton to be there with us on Christmas Day. God answered our prayer. There will never be another Christmas like my Lawton's last Christmas.

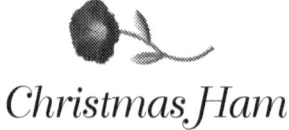

Christmas Ham

Even though there was a lot of hubbub before Christmas, it was a very quiet and peaceful day. Lawty came with his children, Jennings and Kendall. We simply spent time together talking about Christmases past and enjoying one another.

And of course, what would Christmas be without the Christmas ham? On Christmas Eve, there was a knock on the door. It was one of our dear friends who had a burden on his heart and a wonderful talent for cooking. Buddy B heard we were having a crowd for Christmas, and he wanted to provide dinner for us. And provide he did. The feast included a huge yummy ham with all the fixings and a special family recipe apple pie.

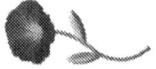

Christmas and Our Pastor

I was very concerned that almost all of our church staff would be out of town during the Christmas and New Year holiday. Who would be here to take care of us if the Lord came for my Lawton? With the seriousness of Lawton's condition and feeling overwhelmingly alone, I sent word to our Pastor about my anxious heart and concern over not being able to reach a pastor should the need arise. We found comfort in his response as he assured us he would come back immediately if Lawton took a turn for the worse or died.

The Lord is my shepherd, I shall not want. (Ps. 23:1)

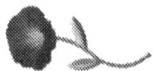

Cathy and Dale's Visit

It was the end of December, and we awaited the arrival of my niece Cathy and her new husband, Dale. We had never met him. They were married in mid-November, which was the same day Cathy learned of her father's death.

I had been cleaning and generally straightening up the house when I noticed a leak under the sink only moments before Cathy and Dale were due to arrive. Knowing my Lawton did not need to be concerned about it, I prayed the Lord would send someone to fix it. As the doorbell rang, I was mopping up the water and debris from under the sink.

It was a happy arrival with hugs in the hall and introductions. My first question to Dale was, "Do you hug?" Then I gave him an "Auntie Jaca" hug.

My second question was, "Are you handy?"

"What do you need?" he asked. He immediately assessed the situation, and within an hour the problem was solved. This was just one more time God came through.

We had a lovely visit getting to know our new nephew and enjoying our time together. It's always fun to be with Cathy. She is unique, loving, funny, and dear to my heart.

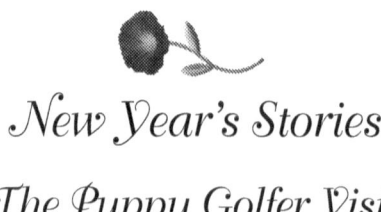

New Year's Stories

The Puppy Golfer Visit

In early December 2001, Troy, one of the puppy golfers from North Carolina, called to announce the birth of his bouncing baby boy Brodie. How proud he was of his boy. He was popping with pride when he talked to my Lawton. It was then the talk started of the Puppy Golfers coming to visit with us in early January 2002. Many details were worked out, and we prayed my Lawton would be well enough to enjoy the Puppies.

They arrived on Friday, January 4 and left on Sunday, January 6.

I cannot tell you how those young men ministered to our hearts. My Lawton absolutely thrived on every moment with them. There was Troy (T-Roy), Andy (Andrew-Belew), Sam (Steady-on Sam), and Dick. They didn't know what to expect when they walked in, because Lawton had a rather difficult day. There was some pain, some nausea, and he was just generally not well. As my Lawton walked into the living room to greet his special guests, it was a precious moment. The reunion was sweet. Hugs were abundant. We all laughed, cried, talked at the same time. How wonderful it was for these great guys to come.

The people from church made certain all of our meals were provided. I didn't really have to lift a finger. The Body of Christ never ceases to amaze me. Everyone was so encouraged and in awe that these men would come to see my Lawton. What a tribute to him their visit was.

We enjoyed a feast on Friday evening. They were amazed the entire meal was provided by our friends. Together we shared much laughter, reminiscing, and general guy talk about golf, sports, work, and family. Lots of pictures of their children were passed around. The Puppy Golfers went to their hotel around 11:00 the first night. On Saturday after breakfast my Lawton wanted to show them around our community. They wanted to go to the real cigar-manufacturing store in Ybor City. After all, it was their tradition to have the finest cigars on the golf course—absolutely a guy thing!

I was so nervous letting my Lawton get in the car with the Puppies. He hadn't been out of my sight for months. I cried when they pulled away from the curb. Oh, did they have a grand time. Lawton showed them his golf clubhouse and course, our church, and of course, the cigar factory. They shared laughter, bantering, kidding, hugs, and admiration.

Their former boss, Mike, had just relocated to Jacksonville with the company, and he was invited to join us for lunch. Mike was the one who contacted Lawton to see if he was interested in working for him in North Carolina. As it turned out, this was truly a special time with these wonderful guys.

Sunday morning came all too quickly. As they came to say their good-byes to my Lawton, I asked my favorite and now standard question, "What was the best part of your visit with us?"

T-Roy said, "Seeing Lawton walking through the bedroom doorway when we arrived."

Andrew Belew said, "The bantering back and forth ... hearing Lawton's humor."

Sam and Dick both said it was the outing and sightseeing the day before.

We all sat there with tears in our eyes, knowing it was the last time we'd all be together with our Lawton. What a treasured memory for all of us. Here are some words that I received in an e-mail from T-Roy's wife not too long ago:

> Troy thinks of Lawton often, especially when they plan their golf trips. He said he feels as if Lawton is with them when they go. There has always been a butterfly or a bird that stays with them the whole time they play their rounds of golf. Troy said that has never happened before. He said he feels like Lawton's spirit is with them.

The Visits to Dr. Zervos

Dr. Zervos was a very intimate part of that time in our lives together. His knowledge, ability to reassure and comfort us and his skill making my Lawton comfortable were a rare gift to us. Throughout all of our hospital stays, he was with us and available even in the wee-small hours of the morning. If he was going out of town, he always made arrangements for Lawton's care. The way he cared for my Lawton will always be an unbelievable memory to me. Dr. Zervos would sit eye-to-eye with Lawton when we talked about the hard stuff. Otherwise, Dr. Zervos would stand by Lawton's bed. Whenever he'd come in and I had my notepad full of questions, he'd always sit with me, answering each one, explaining and even drawing diagrams if I needed clarification. The sensitivity with which he brought the ever difficult news to us is without a doubt the strongest characteristic of his practice. He is a brilliant, highly skilled, and gifted doctor.

Every two weeks we had an appointment with Manny. Lawton looked forward to the visits even though it took great effort for him to prepare and go. He always enjoyed seeing Manny. I think it was the great big hugs that made the visits special.

Our hearts were forever bonded during one of our office visits in January. Rarely do physicians open the door to their heart like Manny did to us. It was very unusual for us to have to wait to see him, but that day we did. Finally, we were called back to a consultation room and waited even more. My Lawton, Mary Jane and I thought it most unusual for him to keep us waiting. We could hear his voice up and down the hall as he saw other patients.

Finally the door opened and in he came, giving Lawton a big hug. Right behind him was a beautiful young woman carrying a rather large tote bag on her shoulder. As Manny introduced his wife, Stella, to us, out popped the head of their dog Barkley. Manny's words were precious, "Lawton, this is my dog Barkley. He brings me great joy and comfort. I thought you'd enjoy him too." Mere words cannot describe how much we were moved by that extraordinary act of kindness. His secretary told us later he had been planning this visit for weeks.

Each one of us was affected by that memory. We often talked about that office visit. Lawton was only able to make it to the office a few more times after the Barkley visit. I'll always treasure and share this beautiful story. I am eternally grateful to Manny for his true affection for my Lawton.

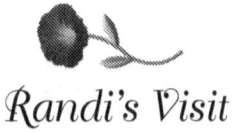

Randi's Visit

Major's daughter Randi is a very special young woman that is always full of life. She is loving, kind, and sensitive, and she went out of her way to visit us. It was January when she and a friend came. They were on their way to New Orleans in their broken-down old car. Of course, all of Randi's earthly possessions were in that car, including her rather large dog. Neither she nor her friend had any money to speak of, yet she wanted to see my Lawton. They stayed with Lynn, Randi's sister, but spent a great deal of time here with us.

Randi's voice and attitude were so tender when she sat across from us at the dining room table, reaching out her graceful hand and said to my Lawton, "If I could fix you, take your pain, or do anything to make you well, I would. I'm so sorry that you are so sick."

We shared with her that we were exactly where God wanted us to be. "This experience was exactly what God wanted for us. His plan is always perfect. He really loves us, and God loves you too, Randi. His love will never change."

Even though Randi is a spiritual person, and even though we talked to her about the Lord and how to know for certain you can spend eternity in heaven with Him, she carries the burden of guilt of poor choices and decisions in her life. She told me she thinks often about the things I've told her and that she prays. Someday, in God's time, she'll understand. I pray it's soon.

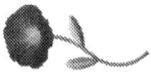

Lauren, Bob, Lexi, and Christian Visit

Each January my niece Lauren (Major's daughter) and her family come to Florida on vacation. They always find time to visit with us. How we enjoyed the visit that year.

Lexi was growing so fast and is very bright. We made the mistake of telling our grandson Jennings this. As soon as she walked in the door, Jennings was challenging her with questions to see if she truly was smarter than he was. With a three-year age difference, Jennings was secure in his challenge. Needless to say, she was a bit intimidated but held her own with him.

And Christian, towheaded as can be, was into everything all the time. Of course he had no idea who we were or why he was here. He just wanted to play with the toys, light the candles, and do boy things.

Lynn's Good-bye to Lawton

My niece Lynn (Major's stepdaughter) lived close by and called one afternoon wanting to know if she could drop by. She sounded very focused and obviously had something on her heart she wanted to share. Her visit blessed us, because for some time she had wanted to tell my Lawton how much he meant to her. She wanted to tell him how his knowledge of so many things helped her and her husband, Jim, decide to move to the Brandon area. I know it was difficult, but she sincerely shared her good-bye and how she appreciated Lawton's help, hospitality, advice, and encouragement as they investigated the possibility of relocating from Chicago.

Lynn and I reflected about this visit after Major died. She said she had asked Major the best way to talk to Lawton about how she felt and how to say good-bye. She wanted to know we would be open to a conversation she desired to have with Lawton.

Lynn beautifully describes in the following pages how she felt during this time.

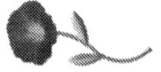

Tommy and Cindy's Visit

Several times throughout Lawton's illness my nephew Tommy would call. Tommy, Fielding's third son, lived in Pennsylvania. He worked in the World Trade Center for months, but on 9/11 he was sick and did not go to work. It was a huge emotional impact for him, losing his co-workers in the attack that day. In February he called us to say he and his fiancée would be heading down to Daytona for the races and wanted to visit with us. It was a good visit. They stayed overnight and we were delighted they would include us in their trip. To this day

Tommy has so much anger at life that has built over the years, but I believe his heart was touched by the genuine love in our home and the honesty we shared about life and dying. Tommy lost both his parents fourteen months apart, but here he saw a different portrait of dying. He certainly heard the Truth spoken during his time with us.

Other family members that were unable to come would call often. I treasured these sweet conversations with Fielding's sons Bobby and Jeff as well as Bobby's daughter Angela. I talked about how Lawton was feeling, how God continued to bless our remaining time together, and all of the ways He touched our lives. The family wanted to understand how we could have such peace during this sad time. As best I could I told of God's perfect plan for our life and how much God's love means. I explained how He comforts everyone who asks Him to be Lord of his/her life.

Our family was drawn to us during this time. To this day it is my prayer they might reflect on this time and choose the Lord as their source of peace.

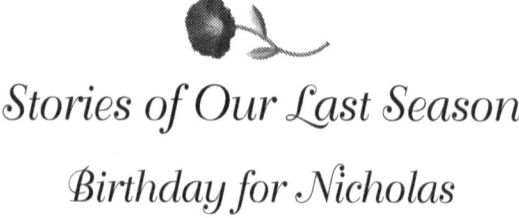

Stories of Our Last Season

Birthday for Nicholas

Our grandson Nicholas wanted his grandpa to live until his twelfth birthday February 14. Fran, Bob, and Nicholas traveled six hours almost every weekend to be with their grandpa. Nicholas was not only losing Lawton but his paternal grandfather as well. Nicholas lived with his Papaw who had experienced several surgeries too.

As my Lawton's illness progressed, the health of Nicholas' Papaw failed quite rapidly. He was moved to a hospital in Atlanta and died one month before my Lawton.

When Nicholas expressed his hope Papaw Lawton would live for his birthday, it became our prayer he live long enough to celebrate it. How faithful is our God. Nicholas thought we forgot all about his birthday. We hid the balloons and special requested ice cream cake that Nicholas wanted. During his birthday dinner celebration we teased him that I did not bake him a cake. We shared the hilariously tragic results of my limp attempts at baking. Fran took great delight in humiliating me with her childhood memories of failed birthday cake stories. Disappointed, Nicholas retreated to his video games. Quickly, we lit the candles on the cake, brought the balloons out of the closet, got Grandpa to the table and watched Nicholas' face as we called him back into the dining room. Everyone was laughing so hard. Nicholas kept saying, "I *knew* you'd have this for me! I just *knew* it!" It was such fun.

Glory be to God for fulfilling this boy's hope.

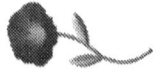

Removing Bushes from the Front of the House

One weekend we decided to open up the front of the house by removing some bushes. We thought it a good plan to move them from the front entryway since I would soon be by myself. Having the front door totally visible from the street was a good idea.

The next weekend when Fran and her husband, Bob, came, they brought a huge chain. And I mean huge. Bob is a contract home builder so he has access to all kinds of equipment and knows a lot about construction. He knew just how to yank those bushes out of the ground. He backed his truck into the front yard, wrapped that mega-chain around one of the bushes and put ruts in the lawn pulling it out. We thought the roots went clear under the house and feared the house would collapse. Of course my Lawton supervised the entire project to make sure it was done correctly. He was so weak, but he didn't want to miss a thing, and he didn't.

The entire neighborhood came out to see what was happening. All the activity and Lawton on the front porch posed an opportunity to visit. Our friend Sandy even took a few of the bushes for her yard. She has a green thumb … I don't. Her bushes are thriving now.

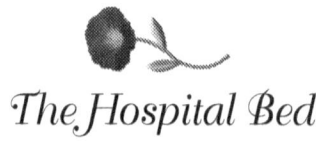

The Hospital Bed

Only a few short weeks before the Lord came for my Lawton, it was decided he would be much more comfortable in a hospital bed. Arrangements were made for delivery the next day.

We needed to move the furniture so it would fit in our bedroom rather than in the family room or some other room that would not be private or comfortable. Several days before we had a call from church letting us know if we needed anything to please call. We knew this anyway, but it was comforting to have that confirmation. We made the phone call the day of delivery and as only God can do, within the hour there were three young men knocking on our door. They had the furniture moved and shortly thereafter the hospital bed was delivered.

In all the activity of the afternoon, I tried hard to remember the names of these young men, but having not written their names down, the information was impossible to retain. When I called the church to thank them for such a quick response, they told me two minutes after my request, they received a call from these young men to volunteer their services for any needs that might arise.

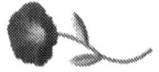

How Many Hot Chocolates Can You Drink in a Night?

Lawton and I developed a ritual of having midnight hot chocolate. After our absolutely anointed prayer time that usually began at midnight or later or after short night-time naps, Lawton would wake me asking for some hot chocolate. You could always tell how his night was by the number of mugs in the kitchen sink come daybreak. Many nights we were alone during our hot chocolate time. But often, depending on who was visiting, others would join in the fun. My sister Major would really get into it, even to the point of adding popcorn or some other tasty treat. Sometimes we were up three or four times a night, sometimes only once, but it was almost every night. These were special times, because my Lawton was usually feeling pretty good in the wee hours of the morning, and he felt like talking.

Our conversations flowed deeply and lovingly. This was part of God's gift of time and grace. We talked often about our journey.

"Babe, how do you think God will use this experience in my life?"

Lawton would respond, "Don't know, Sweet Pea. He'll certainly use it."

"Do you think He'll use me to walk alongside others who will be on the same type of journey?" I would ask.

"Could be," he would say.

How I treasured his wisdom. One night I asked, "Babe, what do you want me to do for the rest of my life?"

"Anything you want," was his reply.

"Well, I know that. But if I knew what you wanted me to do, it would help me in making decisions."

He thought for a moment or two, "I'd like to see you stay in the house as long as you are comfortable. It's a good house, and you'll be safe here. I'd like to see you go on some mission trips if you'd like. You keep talking about it."

We marveled at the kind, encouraging words others would share with us. They told us how strong we were, how open we were, how comfortable we made them feel as we openly talked about his journey to heaven. Often we talked about how people could see God's bubble of peace that surrounded us. We couldn't see it, although we knew it was there. We were simply taking it one step at a time, one day at a time. We were ordinary people, trusting God for each moment together. Someone would visit and perhaps give us a special little book of devotions or encouragement. I would read to Lawton in the wee hours of the night. It brought comfort to us both.

In our midnight prayers we'd pray conversationally as we held one another's hands. As one of us finished, we would squeeze the other's hand. Sometimes, I couldn't tell if he was organizing his thoughts to continue praying or if he had drifted off to sleep. I'll never forget one night when he was so weak he kept drifting in and out of sleep during our prayer. I'd keep squeezing his hand or kissing his cheek. Finally he continued his prayer, "God, I'm sorry. I'm really tired right now. Can I get back to you in a little while? I just need to take a little nap." I don't think God minded.

Planning Lawton's Celebration of Life Service

Sometime in the middle of January, we thought we should start talking to our pastor about Lawton's service. Lawton and I spent some of our hot chocolate conversations about the message and legacy he wanted to leave to his family. We invited our pastor over so he could guide us through this time. His words were so comforting as he shared scripture. Lawton talked about his favorites, his children and what encouragement he wanted to share with family and friends through God's word.

We contacted the funeral home and a representative came to visit. Lawton was focused on what he wanted. He wanted to see up close and personal what would be needed. In a day or so, Lawton gathered enough strength, and off we went to the funeral home to see the urns and all necessary items. He made his selections. As difficult and sad as this process was it was a gift to be able to openly share with him what he wanted and make these decisions together. He needed to know each detail.

The urn he chose was beautiful. It had room for engraved scripture on the four-sided base. Of course Lawton took full advantage of that. He spent days studying scripture, praying and talking to everyone about exactly what he wanted to say. When I said "every detail," I truly meant it. He even selected the font. We faxed the final copy to the funeral home one day before Lawton died.

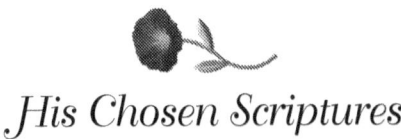

His Chosen Scriptures

Jesus Loves Me, this I know

For God so loved the world, that He gave His only begotten Son, that whoever believes in Him should not perish, but have eternal life. (John 3:16)
My sheep hear My voice, and I know them, and they follow Me; And I give eternal life to them, and they shall never perish; and no one shall snatch them out of My hand. (John 10:27–28)

And I will dwell in the house of the Lord forever. (Psalm 23:6b)

Let not your heart be troubled; believe in God, believe also in Me.
In my Father's house are many dwelling places; if it were not so, I would have told you; for I go to prepare a place for you.
And if I go and prepare a place for you, I will come again, and receive you to Myself … (John 14:1–4)

I have called you by name; you are Mine!
When you pass through the waters, I will be with you … (Isa. 43:1–2)

And He shall wipe away every tear from their eyes; and there shall no longer be any death; there shall no longer be any mourning, or crying, or pain … (Rev. 21:4)

Be anxious for nothing, but in everything by prayer and supplication with thanksgiving let your requests be made known to God. And the peace of God, which surpasses all comprehension, shall guard your hearts and your minds in Christ Jesus.
Finally, brethren, whatever is true, whatever is honorable, whatever is right, whatever is pure, whatever is lovely, whatever is of good repute, if there is any excellence and if anything worthy of praise, let your mind dwell on these things.
The things you have learned and received and heard and seen in Me, practice these things; and the God of peace shall be with you. (Phil. 4:6–8)

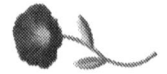

His Grace Is Sufficient

Many times when Lawton was sleeping I would curl up in my Jesus chair. My Jesus chair was in a quiet spot of our home. It was a place I could be by myself, have my devotional books, prayer books, soft music, and generally be with Jesus with no distractions.

As I listened to praise and worship music, I would hear God's heartbeat. I'd voice all of my fears and my gratitude for the time He had given us. I'd talk to Him about how peaceful my husband's face looked as he slept. I'd pray for Lawton's appetite to increase. I prayed his pain would decrease. I prayed our life together would be blessed. I would rest in the bubble of perfect peace God had so gently placed us. The Lord would tell me how much He loved us, and how He would bless each and every moment we had remaining together. It was as if

His glory filled every corner of our home and every crack in my breaking heart. He gave me grace for the next breath. He held me close as I watched Lawton sleep. His sleep was so deep, but it hardly looked like he was breathing at all. I watched him closely. Sometimes I would lie down beside him, hold him gently, and weep with him.

A friend who went through a very difficult and tragic experience with her husband would sign her notes "Swimming in His Marvelous Grace." That was always such a beautiful image, and I marveled at her strength. Sitting there in my Jesus chair, I finally understood what she meant. I too was swimming in His marvelous grace.

Family Pictures

Lawton decided he wanted a picture memory board. This meant pouring over a lifetime of family photos and slides.

For at least two weekends we sorted through every picture in our possession. What fun we had telling stories and joking. There were the bazillion pictures of lakes, single azalea blossoms, turtles on rocks, and forty-five pictures of a cardinal sitting in the evergreen tree we planted in the backyard of our Connecticut condo.

The grandchildren laughed and laughed at their parents—the clothes, the hair styles, and especially Fran's red Patten leather boots. Memories are wonderful things. Don't ever miss an opportunity to talk about special times.

My friend Judy was immersed in scrap booking, so we invited her to assemble the photographed memories. She did a quick sample and brought it over to get Lawton's opinion. We all loved it and even gave her more pictures to work with. We also gave her the freedom to design it any way she wanted, only telling her to listen to the Lord's direction. She brought it over the morning after he died. It was perfect.

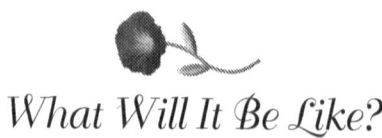

What Will It Be Like?

Often we talked about what it would be like when Jesus came for him. "Lawton, will you tell me when you see Jesus if you can? I mean, will you tell me when He comes for you?"

"If I can I will. I might be in a coma, but I'll try to tell you."

Lawton had begun to pray, "Lord, I know you are coming for me soon. If you take me during the night while Jaca is sleeping, please prepare her heart when she wakes up and I'm gone. Help her to be strong. I want to ask you to make my death quick, and I don't want it to hurt, and Father, could you make it soon?"

My response would be, "Precious Lord, please don't take him while I'm asleep. I want to be by his side, kissing his forehead, and telling him I love him."

We were given a daily devotional book. One night I suggested we skip ahead to see what the devotion would be for Lawton's birthday. It really pierced our heart. It began with this scripture:

> Patient endurance is what you need now, so you will continue to do God's will. Then you will receive all that He has promised. (Heb. 10:36)

Lawton tried so hard to memorize the scripture. With the medications and weakness, it was difficult for him to concentrate. We went over it and over it word by word and phrase by phrase until he had the verse hidden in his heart. My Lawton was living this scripture.

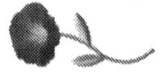

Lawty Gets to Go Home

After months of staying in hotels, rooming with other guys, and spending weekends with us, Lawty was finally allowed to move back into his home. His soon-to-be ex-wife had at long last moved to her own apartment leaving behind a mess in the house. It was awful. My Lawton wanted to help his son move home. I was absolutely against the trip since he still needed meds and monitoring on a regular schedule. He announced on the way home from a visit with Manny he wanted to go.

It was a three hour drive over and a three hour drive back. Even though Mary Jane and Aunt Ruby were with us, I knew no one else would be driving and I really was not looking forward to it. Try as I might, I could not talk him out of it.

As it turned out, it was the most touching thing I have ever witnessed. To watch my Lawton sitting on the floor as weak as he was, washing his son's windows brought tears to our eyes. It was such an expression of love and an everlasting gift to his son. Mary Jane, Aunt Ruby, Kirk and another high school friend Mark and I cleaned bathrooms, kitchen, closets, carpets, and whatever we could do to make it home again for Lawty.

The Coconut Crème Pie Story
(2:00 AM two weeks before he died)

"Babe, you awake?" Lawton wanted to know.

"I am now. What do you need?" was my sleepy reply.

"Nothing, but do we have any coconut crème pie?"

"No, how about some hot chocolate?"

"No. I know it's crazy, but I really want some coconut crème pie. Could you call that place and see if they have any?"

"You do realize that it's two o'clock in the morning, don't you?"

"Yeah, but I really do want it."

"Okay, I'll call. Hi, you don't have any coconut crème pie, do you?"

The gentlemen at the other end of the phone said, "Yes, we do."

Surprised, I responded, "Oh, you do. Okay, how late are you open?"

I was thinking they would be closing any moment but he said, "Twenty-four hours on weekends."

Oh, twenty-four hours a day on Friday and Saturday. Okay, I'll be right down. Don't sell that pie!"

Then Lawton beginning to feel a little guilty and at the same time quite convincing that he really wanted that pie said, "Babe, I'm sorry, but I really do want it."

"I know. It's no problem."

"I'll go with you."

"I think not. What if something happens to you? What would I do in the middle of the night in the middle of Brandon? No. You stay here, and I'll be right back."

That was the best coconut crème pie either of us had ever had. We each ate two pieces. The following morning Mary Jane was mad at us for not waking her up—as if we *could* wake her. We all laughed at that story so much. I can't tell you how many coconut crème pies were brought to us after telling this story. Coconut crème pie was his absolute favorite. Who could have denied getting it for him? He got anything he asked for.

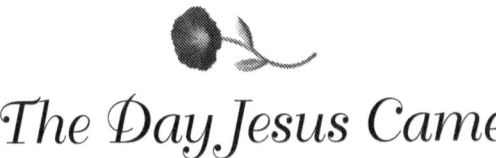

The Day Jesus Came

It was an ordinary, routine day. Over my objections, Lawton insisted he wanted to drill holes in my flower pots I bought a few days before. He wanted the electric drill. He was driven to do this one thing for me. Hardly able to hold the drill, he managed to put a couple of drainage holes in both of the pots. It took every bit of energy he had to accomplish this task. For the remainder of the afternoon, he napped.

Soon it was dinner time. Mary Jane and I prepared a tasty dinner for him. With great difficulty and with my help, he managed to come to the table. Unable to catch his breath, I suggested it might be a good idea for him to lie back down.

Once in bed, his shortness of breath continued. Mary Jane called Hospice and Joy. With her by our side, I prayed for the Lord to give him his breath. In the blink of an eye, Lawton's breathing was normal. We rejoiced, thanking God for answering our prayer and amazed at His goodness.

Just as quick, Lawton was once again unable to breathe. We all knew in that instant Jesus was there for my Lawton, taking him home.

I looked deep into Lawton's eyes and asked if Jesus was there. He couldn't speak. His look said it all. Yes, Jesus was there. I was by his side. I told him I loved him. And Mary Jane kissed his forehead.

Then he was gone. Our prayer was answered.

Thou hast granted me life and loving kindness; and Thy care has preserved my spirit. (Job 10:12)

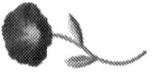

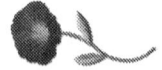

The Beginning of the "Beyond Days"

The Lord's mercy kept me even closer in the bubble of peace. It's a place you can't really describe. Nothing seemed real or on level ground. I put one foot in front of the other as I entered the "beyond days"—the days without my Lawton.

People came to our home. Family arrived from all over. I did things around the house that were automatic. At times I was able to climb in the arms of Jesus and talk or write in my journal to Him. Even though I don't remember writing them, they are a reflection of my heart in the beginning days of my *beyond*:

> Monday, March 18, 2002 is the day we had Lawton's celebration of life service at Bell Shoals Baptist Church. It was a wonderful service, and he would have been so pleased. Many people came. Simeon, our Minister of Music, did a wonderful job singing "Where Grace Abounds." And beautiful "Promise", a women's ensemble, blessed all of us in worship with the family favorite "In the Garden." The Twenty-third Psalm performed by Michael and Linda Adler on their CD and signed by Sue Johnson was a very special, beautiful moment.
>
> When Debbie spoke about our trip to London and Lawton's role as one of the caravan leaders, it was awesome and touched so

many hearts. No one can present the gospel and Jesus as beautifully as she does.

Both Gary Payne and John Russell brought strong messages full of love for my Lawton and our precious Lord. God was glorified in that praise and worship service.

Art Hallett, a dear friend who ministered to us throughout Lawton's illness, offered to sing. Art has a unique way of making songs extensions of his own heart. He's known to add his own twist by changing the words to magnify the Lord. It was a powerful song sung with a powerful voice. It touched hearts and brought tears as we imagined the welcome to heaven Lawton received. The title alone "Welcome To Heaven, My Child" paints a beautiful picture of how you might anticipate leaving this life longing to be in the Lord's presence. Hearing the personal greeting from him upon arrival in heaven, "You have run the race, you have kept the faith." My heart weeps with joy when I imagine my Lawton's first glimpse of the gates of pearl and streets of gold. Ah, what a Savior.

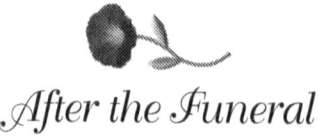

After the Funeral

Immediately after the funeral, during a reception at church, we were greeted by so many friends with hugs and thoughtful words. Soon we were home. It was just the family sharing sadness and beginning to put the pieces back together.

When my sister Major left that evening, my heart broke even more. Her cancer had returned, and she was beginning her second round of chemotherapy. She faced a big hill to climb.

Journal Reflections

It's Tuesday, March 19 and everyone left today. Mary Jane will stay with me until after Easter. I know the Lord prepared my heart for the time she would go home.

Awoke early this Wednesday morning. Heart is heavy today. The task for today is to write notes of thanks to folks who have ministered to us during Lawton's illness and home going. I know the tears will flow as I remember how their acts of kindness and love touched our hearts and encouraged us.

Easter. Our church moved to the Florida State Fairgrounds for a beautiful Easter service of just under 5,000 people. The Lord touched my heart with Debbie's prayer about the members of our church family who were severely injured in a recent terrorist attack at a church in Pakistan. Debbie told us how He is guiding them down the road to recovery. Mary Jane and I shared a delightful dinner with Linda and Jeff. They have been so good to all of us throughout Lawton's illness and home going and they are so precious to my heart.

It's nighttime, and my heart is so very heavy. Mary Jane left this morning, and today was my first day back at work, Monday April 1, 2002. The corner is turned.

I talked to Major (she had her second chemo treatment today, which was five hours for the infusion). Other friends and family called to check on me.

I had a good, long, deep cry when I got home from work. This was my first time coming into an empty home. I tried to go to bed early (it's now 9:32 PM). Thought it might help to put my heart in print. The Lord is molding me and holding me. I am so tired. I am so sad. I really miss my Lawton.

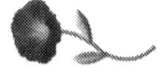

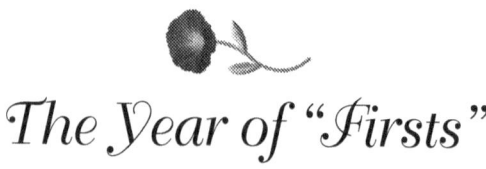

The Year of "Firsts"

My Lawton and I had time to talk about so many things, and among them was what I would do on the special days—birthday, anniversary, Thanksgiving, Christmas, and others. We came up with some things we thought would be good for me, encouraging and not too sad without him by my side. Here is what God planned for me.

The First Birthday/Wedding Anniversary Celebration

Our anniversary was the first big hurdle after Lawton's death. It seemed like a good idea thirty-one years ago to get married on my birthday, but this year it was really painful. No one wanted me to be alone, and so it was.

On Friday everyone gathered at a nearby restaurant for a wonderful time of remembering and celebrating. They planned something very special. Each one of the thirty guests brought a beautiful silk flower and presented it to me with a hug. Everyone whispered sweet words of love, encouragement, and blessing in my ear. We laughed and cried. Each time I look at those beautiful flowers arranged in the stunning vase they gave me, I am reminded of the Body of Christ. Each person is unique and gifted with different attributes of Christ. When the individual flower is added to the others I see a beautiful portrait of our Lord. It's my very own "Bouquet of Christ." I continue to thank this very special group for making this day so very precious for me. When people comment on the huge and lovely flower arrangement that adorns my dining room table, I tell them this story and remember anew the love shared with me that day.

There were more flowers, cards, balloons, and of course, the ever-present chocolate.

Lawty sent flowers to the office for me. It took my breath away. He simply signed the card "Lawton."

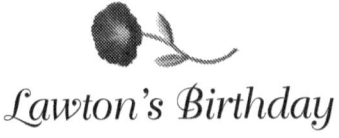

Lawton's Birthday

Celebrating what would have been Lawton's sixty-fifth birthday, I planned all year to have a special, private time at the end of the day to spend remembering my Lawton. I knew precious Linda would remember this day. We met for lunch. We remembered my guy, cried, laughed, told stories, talked about days past, and the days to come. She wanted to know what I was doing in the evening, so I told her my plan. I had kept one slice of last year's birthday cake, and it was for this special night. I was going to eat that cake no matter how terrible it tasted, listen to Josh Groban's "*To Where You Are,*" talk to my Lawton, and gratefully thank God for the time we had together.

Thanksgiving

I spent the first Thanksgiving with Lawty, his children, and his friend Bernie. Bernie wanted to make the day special not only for Lawty but for me as well. She graciously welcomed me into her home. It was beautiful, comfortable, open, and inviting. I met her sons. Soon it was time for Lawty to pick up his children Jennings and Kendall. He would be gone almost two hours. During the time Bernie and I were alone we talked about my Lawton. I was thankful for her kindness and sensitivity. She shared things about Lawty's journey of grief and how they both appreciated my words of encouragement to him.

After Jennings and Kendall arrived we had great fun watching them ride up and down the street on the little moped and watching the hilarious attempts at shooting baskets with a basketball ten times too big for Kendall.

The meal was wonderful. All of the traditional Thanksgiving touches were there with the exception of the rolls, which turned out hard as rocks. I quickly called them the "rockin' rolls." Everyone thought that was funny, and from that point on, we all enjoyed the "rockin' rolls" and the feast.

Christmas

Not having a plan is not a good plan. Lawton and I could not decide what I should do the first Christmas after his death. As much as I tried to develop a plan, nothing would come. I sought God's plan for this day, but I didn't know what He wanted me to do. I thought I would serve meals to the homeless in the Tampa Port at the Seamen's Ministry. I knew I didn't want to have people here. I didn't want to decorate or cook or bake. I didn't want to do anything.

My sister Major wanted me to come up to Charlottesville and be with all of her family. As much as I wanted to go, I simply could not do it. There would be so many people there, and I just didn't think I could cope. This was Major's Christmas, and it was magnificent for her. The Lord would give her only one more Christmas, and she needed to be with her family.

I felt I needed to stay home. I wanted to be in my sanctuary.

Prior to Christmas I enjoyed shopping for everyone, going to all of the parties, and participating in the festivities. When it came time to wrap and give the many gifts I had bought, I simply could not bring myself to do it. I didn't want to see the presents. I didn't want to have Christmas. I wanted it to go away. Finally I agreed to go to Lawty's on Christmas Day and to pick up my grandchildren on the way. I planned to spend the night there with all of them. Had I not made this commitment and had they not depended on me to deliver the children, I would have pulled the covers over my head and spent the entire day in bed ignoring Christmas and praying for it to be gone. The memories of our last Christmas together were still extremely fresh in my mind.

We arrived at Lawty's home, and the children excitedly tore into all of their gifts. It was a normal Christmas with wrapping paper flying, laughter at the delight in their voices, and more laughter at their disappointment with the packages containing socks or underwear.

I held back tears when Lawty served our traditional Christmas dinner complete with Cornish hens. I remembered our very first Christmas as a new family so many years ago in Connecticut when I prepared Cornish hens for everyone. It was like your own personal child-sized turkey. The kids loved it. They had their own leftover "turkey."

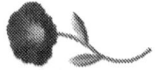

The Next Big Day—Valentine's Day

I really hadn't given much thought to Valentine's Day although I knew it would be a sad day. However, some very dear people planned something special. My friendship with Tricia and Bill had grown over the last several months. I selected Bill as my financial advisor. Admiring this couple since I met them years before, I knew I could depend on them and trust everything they said. I had no idea how significant they would be to me as they slowly adopted me into their family. Eventually Bill would also become my deacon.

Months before Valentine's Day they made me reserve the day. Since I knew them to be fun, loving people, I knew they had a grand surprise. As the day drew near, I wondered what they had planned for me. Reliable sources began to warn me of Bill's addiction to fairs and festivals. For two weeks in February, the Florida State Fair is held in Tampa.

Do you have any idea how much fun you can have at a State Fair with a "Fair Junkie?" Bill is a world-class "Fair Junkie." One would think he lives from fair to fair. We ate "Fair Fries," fudge, funnel cake, and Italian sausage subs. We laughed at the weird chickens and roosters. We marveled at the beautiful quilts and other handcrafted items. We shopped (mostly me) and took advantage of fair specials. It was a grand time, even if they didn't let me go on the big "Bungee Sling."

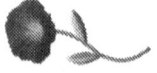

New York on the First Anniversary

My sister Major came for a visit in January. I told her I wanted to go to New York for the first anniversary of Lawton's death, and I wanted her to go with me. She didn't hesitate for a moment. We had planned to go for a long time, and it just seemed like the right thing to do. As usual she procrastinated in getting her airline reservation so the price soared out of reach. She chose to take the train from Charlottesville to Penn Station.

My flight came in long before her train did. The plan was to check into the hotel, meet her at Penn Station, and taxi back to our hotel. When I arrived at the hotel, there was a package waiting for me. I thought it was from the hotel, thinking they somehow knew the significance of our visit. When I got to the room I opened it and discovered it was from our niece Cathy. I decided to wait for Major so we could finish opening it together. Once we did, we discovered mostly chocolate. It was such a thoughtful a gift. She wanted to share this time with us and make it special.

That evening, Wednesday, March 12, we had dinner with my god-father Don, his daughters and grandchildren and longtime family friend Virginia White. Don was our next-door neighbor growing up.

It was an adventure getting to his apartment. Major and I walked many blocks after taking our first subway ride. I guess we got off at the wrong stop or our directions were poor. We met a nice man who gave us good directions, and we eventually found Don's apartment building since we weren't as lost as we originally thought.

At evening's end, on Don's advice, and escort to the bus stop, we took the bus back to the hotel. That was very uneventful, and we could see where we were going.

On Thursday we slept in. We were both so tired. My mood was good, and of course I thought of my Lawton often. This was the one year anniversary of his death.

We met Virginia, a longtime friend of the family, for lunch on the Upper West Side. It was cold, rainy, and a lot like the lunch my Law-ton and I had with Virginia in London two years earlier celebrating our thirtieth anniversary. I reminded her of our visit, and it was a sweet remembrance for both of us.

Taking a bus back to the hotel, we enjoyed the sights and sounds of Manhattan. It took forever. Traffic was terrible due to a water main break along Fifth Avenue. We were re-routed around it into curb-to-curb cars, trucks, buses, and absolute gridlock.

My heart's desire was to see *The Lion King* that day. But we didn't have tickets and were unable to purchase any beforehand since Broadway was on strike. Major and I decided to walk to the theater to see if by some remote chance there were tickets available. During the walk, I was praying these words, "Lord, you know it's my heart's desire to see that play tonight. But I know whatever you have for me will be perfect, and I'm fine with that. But, you know it's my hearts desire to see *The Lion King* tonight, but …" And on it went.

When we arrived at the box office I inquired if tickets were available. His smirk was not encouraging as he asked, "For when?"

"For tonight."

With somewhat of a chuckle he went to look. "I'll see what we have." When he returned, there were tickets in his hand. "Well, we've just had a cancellation, and we have two that are pretty good seats." We both had our credit cards out so fast it was like quick draw. I didn't care if the seats were on the moon. I was getting my heart's desire.

God answered my prayer because our seats could not have been more perfect. We were orchestra left, eighth row, two seats in from the aisle. I simply sat there and wept. I wanted to jump on stage and announce to the world what the Lord had done for me that day. It was absolutely perfect. I needed something beyond belief, something I could feel, taste, hear, and see. I needed something real only God could do. I know without a doubt He took great delight in giving me the desire of my heart.

The next day we enjoyed the Metropolitan Museum of Art with Don. What fun seeing the special exhibits through his eyes. He is an artist himself and great, knowledgeable critic. We enjoyed his comments and opinions on the artwork.

Major and I managed to get half-price tickets for "*Aida*" that evening. The music was outstanding, and it was a beautiful love story. It was another delightful day we were able to spend together. Before we left the next day, I simply had to take a side trip to what was advertised as the world's largest jewelry store. I know no one will believe it, but I didn't buy a thing. Of course Major did.

I thought the tears would be gone once I went to NYC, but that was not the case. Once the plane left the ground I was in tears. They were not sobs—just gentle tears. This was another page in my journey without my Lawton.

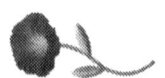

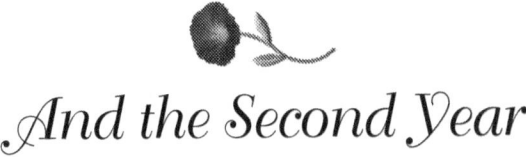

And the Second Year

As the first anniversary was quickly approaching, Pastor Buddy of Benevolence and Hospital, who had spent so much time with us during the hospital days, asked if I would share a brief testimony during our worship services one Sunday. As procedure, the ministerial staff was required to enlist someone to give a brief comment and testimony at the end of each service. Immediately I said no. I wouldn't do it. The Lord, however, had a different plan. As I prayed, He showed me He had been preparing my heart. I should seek His face for the words He wanted me to share. Thirteen months to the day after Lawton died I spoke these words at all three morning worship services:

> I'm sure 9/11 means something different to each one of you. To me, it means seeing God's hand at work through many of you sitting here today. On 9/11 my husband was diagnosed with pancreatic cancer. It was a lot to process in one day.
>
> Within moments of receiving this news, there were powerful prayer warriors immediately surrounding us in our home. From that day I learned how to receive encouragement from the Body of Christ. Our needs were met by Him through you even before my Lawton or I knew there was a need. Each day was a blessing as the Fellowship of Encouragement ministered to us.
>
> We were in and out of the hospital many times during the months that followed. With each procedure, there was someone from our ministerial staff, or a deacon, or one of you by my side. Sometimes it was all of the above.

The Lord gave us incredible gifts during my Lawton's last six months. God healed relationships within our family. He drew us closer to Him as He prepared our hearts for the time when Jesus would take my Lawton home. He took us to a place where grace abounds.

We saw so many, many answers to our prayers and yours. My Lawton and I clung to the promise that God's mercies were new every day. Even today!

It is only through the power of the Risen Savior I can stand here to share with you a part of our story.

This church offers many avenues for you to grow in the Lord. This is a place to find comfort, joy, peace, and hope. No matter your situation, there is someone here who has walked the same path and will walk beside you each step of your journey.

It was a privilege to stand before so many who encouraged us on our journey. As I prayed in preparation of what I would say during the service that day, God also revealed to me an evident need within that body of believers.

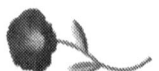

The Visit Back to North Carolina

I knew there would come a time when I would go back to North Carolina to visit those who meant so much during our time there. I also knew it would be a blessing, but never expecting the blessing to be for me. In preparing for the trip, Jackie invited me to stay with her. Debra and Eddie also invited me to stay with them. Since Jackie's husband was deployed to Afghanistan at the time, I thought it would be good for both of us to spend time with one another. It proved to be encouraging for both of us. I always feel welcome in her home. She is such a gracious hostess.

Debra offered to have a luncheon for me after church. "Invite as many as you want—thirty, fifty people. Whoever you want," she said. It was a wonderful time and many came. I was able to visit with the people who made our time in North Carolina so special. Sharing the *Ah-Ha* moment the Lord had given me about our four years in North Carolina was an extraordinary experience.

> God moved us from Brandon and from all that was good. He moved us from the life we built, the church, the friends, and everything. He planted us in an area that was totally different and almost foreign. The reason He did that was for us to grow closer to Him, because that was all we had. It was simply preparation for what lay ahead for us.

I was able to tell them how important they were to us, thank them for embracing us for the season we shared with them, encourage them to keep doing what they were doing, and praying for others.

> And we know that all things work together for good to those who love the Lord to them who are called according to His purpose.(Rom. 8:28)

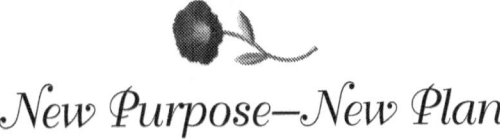

New Purpose–New Plan

As I prayed for His wisdom, I was reading a book so many have been touched by—*The Purpose Driven Life*. Through studying this book and listening to the Lord as He prompted my heart, I realized His plan is about Him, not me. He wanted me to provide a ministry for widows. I began talking to other sister widows to see if that might be something of interest and need within our members. No matter who I talked to, the answer was a resounding yes. I talked about this to my faithful prayer warriors, here and in North Carolina, and my pastor. Everyone encouraged me to proceed.

My deacon at the time, Bill, and his wife, Tricia, were so supportive. Linda and Jeff were instrumental in the development process.

Linda even recruited leadership and wrote to our pastor about the desire embedded in my heart. Scripturally, since the deacon body is a widow's spiritual head, and the deacons serve directly under the pastor, it was only logical this ministry would be structured under our pastor's leadership. Since widows are all ages, not just seniors, developing the ministry under a senior adult ministry was not the answer. The women's ministry was more event and special classes directed for women in all stages of family life. God was directing a pursuit of a ministry specialized and focused on widows.

> Do not call to mind the former things, or ponder things of the past. Behold, I will do something new, now it will spring forth; will you not be aware of it? I will even make a roadway in the wilderness, rivers in the desert. (Isa. 43:18–19)

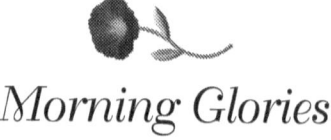

Morning Glories

Several names and scriptures were suggested for the group, but the one that moved my heart was from Jackie in North Carolina.

> Weeping may last for the night, but joy comes in the morning. (Psalm 30:5)

Our name became "Morning Glories."

A dear friend of mine, Mary Dana Hardin is a gifted and accomplished artist. One day I asked her if there was a morning glory in her collection. There wasn't, but she said there was a fence with morning glories in full bloom. I told her about the developing ministry and our need of a logo. She said she would do anything to help, and off she went to take pictures of the morning glories. Mary Dana brought back several beautiful photos of the fence for me to review. Not wanting to make the decision totally on my own, I waited to present the pictures at our first meeting.

A small group of six met in June 2003 to talk, pray, plan, and see if this was a ministry of God, not of Jaca. I didn't know exactly what my role would be. I thought because of my position at the church, it would be natural to be a liaison between the deacons, pastor, and Morning Glories. Everything the Lord gave me I shared with the ladies, and they thought it all wonderful. I gave each one a different book I had received to comfort me through grief. Their assignment was to review it, keeping in mind it might be something we would share with new widows as they began their journey through grief.

We prayed God would show us what He wanted. My specific prayer was to be shut down if we headed in a direction that was not what He wanted. Our plan was to meet again in a few weeks to hear what the Lord had revealed to each of us.

As I had prayed, the Lord shut me down. God had given me so much in the early development of the ministry. After our initial meeting, He did not show His plan to me for the future design of the ministry. I had nothing to contribute at our next meeting. Naturally the women were shocked. I told them, "It's all up to you to fill this blank page we are starting on."

Once they got over the initial jolt, their ideas flooded the room. As I listened to them, I realized what was happening. The Lord wanted them to own this ministry as much as I did. It *was* about Him.

We planned a tea for mid-August. We made personal phone calls to each widow in our membership and every widow who ever visited our church for any reason. Our only plan was to provide an atmosphere of fellowship. We all met new friends, discovered common interests, and just enjoyed the afternoon.

From that beginning, we have frequent luncheons after Sunday worship service and occasional outings to the movies or plays. We have care group leaders who reach out to those in their group. We still don't know all that God is doing with the ministry. We simply take it one day at a time.

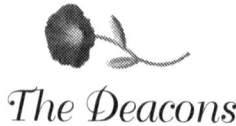

The Deacons

In September 2003, I stood before the deacons in their monthly meeting to introduce the new ministry called Morning Glories. I gave a brief summary of my journey into widowhood. Then I asked these questions of the men:

"First, how many of you are married?" All raised their hands.

"Second, how many of you believe you will live longer than your wife?" Not one raised their hand.

Well, you could have heard a pin drop. Many were looking at me with that deer in the headlights look. Proceeding, I asked more questions giving them time to ponder and write their answers. They didn't need to answer aloud—only on paper or in their hearts.

As I continued, these are some of the things I spoke of:

> I asked the deacons to think about or write down what they believe will be the most important thing their wives will need after they die—
>
> • Immediately—in the first several weeks
>
> • Within the first six months
>
> • Within the first year
>
> My questions to the deacons continued as I wanted them to begin understanding the emotion and needs of a widow. I was hoping that these questions would open dialogue with their wife and help as they partner in ministry to their assigned widow.
>
> • What are some dates that are important to you, your wife, and your family ... Birthdays? Anniversary?
>
> • How do you think she will feel on these days during the first year?

- The second year?

- Have you ever talked about these things?

Since I have been getting together with some of my sister Morning Glories, we have talked about the things we found we needed during the first few weeks.

Friends, family, church family to surround us, pray for us, send notes, hugs—lots of them. Get us out of the house.

It's so easy to just pull the covers over your head and pretend that all will be back to normal when you get up. The fact is nothing will be normal again. Normal is going to be different—different for all of us. It may take years (if ever) to feel normal again.

For me and many of my sister Morning Glories, it was hard and emotional even coming to church. Coming to worship alone for the first time is extremely difficult. Where do I sit? Who do I sit with? Where do I belong? I don't want to impose or intrude on couples.

I didn't even feel like I belonged with our Sunday school class, even though they would have welcomed me with open arms. It would be just too difficult and sad. So many of my sister widows have told me they feel like a fifth wheel or a fish out of water.

I recommend the deacon maintain weekly contact whether by phone, note, home visit, or out for a meal. Be sure that your wife is a part of this time.

At the end of this first meeting with all of the deacons, they gathered around me to pray for me and for the Morning Glories Ministry. They understood what God was doing in and through the ministry. It was a deeply moving time for me to think that the Lord was truly using my journey to comfort and instruct others.

The Morning Glories Ministry is a work in progress. Over the 2004 Christmas holidays, the Lord once again nudged, cradled, and sustained me. He continued to gently reveal that He wanted more for the ministry. Even though I realized it needed to go to the next level, my prayers seemed unanswered.

It was only after the holidays in a conversation with my boss, Ted Badger, I knew without a doubt the direction God was leading. Ted is the Pastor of Single Life Ministries and months earlier had graciously agreed to be the ministry pastor. I knew I could not give the Morning Glories Ministry the structure needed, but Ted could.

Together (it was mostly Ted) we developed the Morning Glories Ministry guidelines. As you look at scripture, it is evident the Lord has a special place in His heart for widows. His mandate is clear to "care for widows who are widows indeed" (2 Timothy 5) Ted brought organization to the ministry, and I brought the heart. As we partnered with our Deacon Fellowship, more needs of widows were recognized and met through the resources of our church.

In developing the guidelines, Ted designed it not only for our church organization but to make it portable to other denominations. We were not reinventing the wheel—just putting it back on the vehicle. I continued to stand in awe at how the Lord used my simple journey to bless me in the "beyond" days.

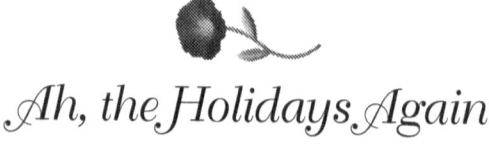

Ah, the Holidays Again

I decided to go to my sister's for Thanksgiving. Everyone was planning to be there including all of her children, some of her stepchildren, our niece Cathy, and her children. Even Mary, who was caregiver for Major's mother-in-law, would be there. Major always made the holidays a special event in her home. She always celebrated with flair and her signature touch. The dining room could seat about twenty or more if we pulled in highchairs for the little ones.

I flew in early in the week and had first pick of the bedrooms, something you always want to do at Major's. We had some good sister time before the deluge of family. I went with her for her weekly chemo treatment, finally meeting those who cared so beautifully for her. And I finally met her "Manny," Dr. Morris. It was evident how much they thought of my sister and admired her determination.

We girls started planning a trip to England in the spring. What fun we had trying to decide all the details. Major was enthusiastically participating in the planning. We were all excited with the possibility of it really happening.

One evening after Major went to bed the nieces, cousins and I started a serious conversation about Major's illness. How were we individually dealing with it? How could we be more supportive of Major? My prayer was to see her family through God's eyes, not mine. As our conversation progressed, the Lord truly let me see into their hearts. Each one was so different, but each one was so sad knowing this might be the last Thanksgiving with Major. I listened to their feelings and delighted they could share so openly about their sadness.

It was such a good Thanksgiving I invited myself back for Christmas.

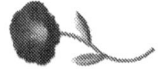

Christmas "Big Girl" Trip

I knew getting flights out of Tampa would be almost impossible as well as expensive. I opted to drive so I would have flexibility in timing, where I went and when. The next few weeks I mapped my route trying to see people all the way up to Virginia and all the way back.

My first stop was in Georgia with Fran and her family. My friend, Miz Pat, rode with me on the first leg. Her son lived about two hours from Fran, so he met us at Fran's home. We went out to dinner that evening and church in the morning. The day was beautiful, so I took advantage of the sunshine and started the next leg of my "big girl" trip. Fran gave me directions to a shortcut for a good portion of my drive that day. My plan was to drive from Warner Robbins to Greensboro. As good as her directions were I still needed my safety net—OnStar. This was a huge asset many times on the trip. I will never leave home without it. Even though I intended to stay in Greensboro, I didn't like the look of the motel I chose. I proceeded to

Danville for the night, then on into Charlottesville the next day. The plan was to meet Major and two of her friends downtown for lunch. They were celebrating a birthday.

Christmas at Major's was full of hugs, gifts, good food, laughter, and children. The tree took days to decorate. Everyone that came participated in adorning the tree.

The Saturday after Christmas, I left to spend the night in Richmond with my Auntie Ann. How I love this woman. She was a pillar of strength, comfort, and understanding, especially since her husband, Charlie, died almost two years before my Lawton. Auntie Ann had a special dinner planned. Her son Bert, daughter Beverly and Beverly's family came.

I left early the next morning so I could make the two hour drive to North Carolina in time to worship at the church Lawton and I attended when we lived in Oxford. What fun it was to surprise them and even more fun to get all of the hugs. After having a long leisurely lunch with Debra, I stayed with Jackie. Her Ed had been home for a brief visit and left the day before to return to Afghanistan. My visit was timely—God's timeliness.

The next day, after stopping to see the Puppy Golfers, I headed south for home. It was a wonderful trip. It was something I wasn't sure I could do all by myself. I said on this trip God was my pilot, OnStar was my navigator, and I just sat there doing the driving and eating all of the wonderful snacks people provided along the way.

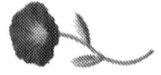

...And They Said ...

Notes from Precious Miz Pat

Whenever trouble comes your way, let it be an opportunity for joy. For when your faith is tested, your endurance has a chance to grow. So let it grow for when your endurance is fully developed, you will be strong in character and ready for anything. (James 1:2^b–4 New Living Translation)

I was a neighbor of Jaca and Lawton. We lived across from each other for a number of years. They had been away for a few years and were back home for just a short time. It was such a happy homecoming and then Jaca began to share that Lawton was not well—just generally not feeling tip-top.

Then there were tests, hints of possible cancer, and the dread news—a diagnosis of a malignancy. There was of course shock, prayers for God's healing touch, and wisdom for the doctors. Through all the pain, there was a prevailing sense of peace and a gentle stirring of love. It was love and trust in God and a heart full of love for each other.

Jaca and Lawton's church family rallied around them showing their love in practical ways and surrounding them with spiritual support. Yes, there were traumatic moments and down times, but through it all, they were enveloped in an awesome prism of God's grace. To have been privileged to share this precious time with Jaca and Lawton, even in a small way, was such a blessing.

—Pat Cameron (spiritual mentor and dear friend)

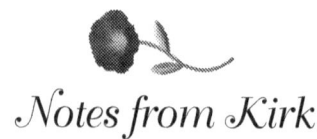

Notes from Kirk

Dear Jaca,

I'd like to share some thoughts and memories I have for Lawton DePriest Sr.

I met Lawton Jr. (Lawty) at Brandon High School, and we soon became best of friends. It wasn't long after when I met my extended family, Lawton Sr. and yourself.

I have great memories of the unselfish time you both shared with me and the Brandon High School wrestling team. Whenever the boys start to reminisce, one story always comes to mind, and that is the weekend in Daytona Beach 1980. I thank you both for letting us be kids and have one of the best times in our lives.

I know more than a couple times you guys would go to sleep and wake up with more people than you expected for breakfast. Thanks for sharing your home and hospitality.

I remember the first time I played golf at a nice country club, Saddlebrook. Even though Jr. and I weren't the best golfers, it was a special treat for Mr. DePriest to include us. He included us a lot. I felt like one of the men. I have a passion for golf that I share with Lawty. And Mr. D helped foster that love. While on the subject of golf, it was very special that Lawton and Lawty decided to give me Mr. DePriest's golf clubs. I have been playing better and more often. There isn't a time I'm on the course I don't think about Mr. DePriest and the awesome gift he gave me.

As a kid, I didn't see a great deal of marriages work out, but seeing you and Mr. DePriest and the love you guys shared, it gave me hope.

Mr. D was always even-tempered, always had kind words, and was very supportive. When Mr. D was diagnosed with cancer, he found the positive. When we were alone one night at the hospital, he told me that cancer gave him an opportunity to say good-bye to all the ones he loved, unlike the people that vanished on September 11, 2001.

I feel my life is better for knowing Lawton DePriest Sr., and I know you feel the same way.

Thank you both for letting me be part of your family.

Love, Kirk

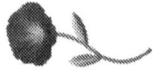

Notes from Central Baptist Church Sunday School Class

We will never forget how your enthusiasm for Central Baptist Church always seemed to grow. You participated as if you had been at Central all of your life, and I often thought what a wonderful gift from God to have sent two energetic people like you to help build up a church. You both were always so helpful and encouraging, and you always had wonderful ideas with so much support.

I can still see the twinkle in Lawton's eyes when he said, "You need to build it big." He always let you know you needed long-term vision, and we will always be so grateful to the two of you for what you contributed then and now.

Thank you from the bottom of our hearts for speaking to us even though you are no longer present with us. We still feel your love and presence as we think of you and your contribution. You truly have been a blessing to us in so many ways, and so many of God's people are and will continue to be blessed because of your commitment to the Lord.

I could go on and on, but hopefully this will tell you how much we appreciated your ministry at Central Baptist Church.

Have a great day, and may God bless you and your ministries.

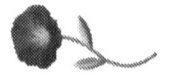

Pat Springer–My Reflection

Lawton … Precious, funny, interesting, charming, encouraging, thoughtful, full of life's experiences (especially when it came to food and the best places to eat). These are some of the things Lawton became to Chuck and me over the years our friendship developed. It didn't matter if jobs caused us to be separated for months or years at a time. When God brought us back together, it was as if no time had passed at all.

It all started when God brought Jaca and me together, knitting our hearts and lives in an extra-special bond. Jaca was ready to continue growing in the Lord and wanted to become active in church while Lawton wasn't in any hurry. After all, Sunday church was hard to fit into his schedule (which was planned around his love of golf). And oh, how he loved golf! But as we prayed, loved, and extended invitations to class socials, little by little God warmed Lawton's heart. He returned to church and put the Lord's work and agenda first in his life. I will never forget the Sunday after years of praying we saw Lawton walk down the aisle of church asking for his membership to be transferred to our church. We knew that meant Lawton was really making a new commitment in his life. He never turned back from this new zeal for the Lord and His church.

I remember how he loved to cook. This was good since Jaca, like myself, sometimes struggles in this area. I can still remember that huge pot of spaghetti he made from a special recipe in a magazine. It was delicious, but it could have fed an army. I still have a copy he gave me, and every time I come across it, I have to smile.

When the time came he started feeling physically bad, I never heard him complain. Even though I know it must have been extremely difficult, he continued to be faithful to as many of his church responsibilities as he could. He was always trying to smile, always encouraging, and always interested in what was going on in other's lives. During those long, drawn-out days of wasting away with a dreadful disease, he continued to share his love and hope in the Lord with whoever was attending to him. When the end of his earthly life got closer and closer, heaven got more real and more real. Without a doubt, as he began to realize more and more it was not the Lord's will to heal him, he began to long for the total healing of heaven. Sure, the thing he hated most was leaving his precious Jaca, but he faced every part of his difficult assignment with grace, strength, and courage, which I believe came from his Lord, Jesus Christ.

My life will forever be blessed by the special friendship of Lawton.

While on earth I continue to miss that twinkle in his eye, his wonderful stories, and that precious bond the Lord built between us. Once a year the most spectacular event in sports takes place in Augusta, Georgia. It's the Masters Golf Tournament. The golf course is glorious with flowers and trees in magnificent colors. Every year as I watch this display on TV I think of the year Lawton realized his dream of being there to see the golf pros and enjoy the excitement of the tournament. Oh, how special this was to him. There are so many little things throughout the year that have a connection with Lawton. They all bring a smile to my face. Thanks Lawton for the memories!

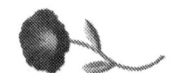

Robert DuBois (and Dora Too)

What do I think of when I think of Lawton? Someone who, even though he has to catch a plane, and the time for departure is getting near, never seemed to be in a hurry. He had a calm spirit that let you know he'd be on time.

Playing golf with him was always enjoyable, and you would never know if he were winning or losing by his outward appearance. It was always the same—cheerful and calm. But when approached off the course (maybe in the concourse) and the subject of golf came up, his eyes would light right up. (This last statement is really from Dora, because she observed both of us enjoying just talking about golf.) Lawton was a kind of "yup" guy. Discuss a subject and his response might be yup, yup, yup, but when it was his turn to respond, you'd find his opinion was very good and probably better than yours which you had just been talking about.

God loves you. Love back.

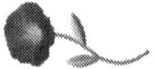

Linda Wells—I Remember Lawton

Lawton DePriest was a very quiet, gentle man. He and his beautiful wife, Jaca, joined our Bible study class in 1987. Lawton was a man of few words, but when he spoke everyone listened. Jaca and I became good friends, and Lawton and Jeff enjoyed playing golf together at Buckhorn Country Club.

Jaca and Lawton moved to North Carolina in 1995. We did not see them again until they moved back to Brandon in the summer of 1999. We were so happy to have them back home.

I remember seeing a very thin Lawton at a church picnic. Jeff and I decided he must be on a diet. A few days later we learned Lawton was ill. So began our journey with two very special friends.

Lawton was diagnosed with pancreatic cancer. He was in for the fight of his life, and fight he did. We were amazed at how he continued to come to church and live as normal a life as he could. The Lord truly girded Lawton with his strength (Psalm 18:39).

There were many visits and prayers at Tampa General Hospital. Jeff and I just wanted to be there. We couldn't do much for Jaca and Mary Jane other than give them plenty of hugs, prayers, and bring them some outside food. It made our hearts hurt to see Lawton suffer so much, but we wanted them to know how much we loved them.

One of my best memories was one afternoon at Lawton and Jaca's home. I was busy in the kitchen (I am a Martha), and Lawton and Jaca were sitting at the dining room table. They were just talking and sharing with each other. They seemed like love-struck teenagers when they looked at each other. How precious that was—how special! Lawton could hardly sit in the chair he was so weak, but he so enjoyed sitting in "his" chair.

Another very special time for me was one afternoon when I dropped by to see Jaca and Lawton for a quick visit. I wanted so badly to help. I just wanted to do something, but there wasn't anything I could do. Lawton was sitting on the sofa in the den by himself. I asked him if I could pray for him. I knelt on the floor by his feet. I wanted so badly for Lawton to live. I remember pleading with God to spare his life if it was His will. The tears flowed from both our eyes. By this time Lawton was a skeleton of the man he once was, but his spirit was stronger than ever. Lawton taught everyone who knew him that a personal relationship with Jesus Christ gives us strength to endure anything in this life.

Jaca is one of my dearest friends. She radiates Christ. It was because of the relationship she and Lawton shared with each other and their close walk with the Lord they were able to live a lifetime together in those few months. They left nothing undone or unsaid.

Jeff and I had never walked this path with friends before. We counted it a privilege and an honor. Jaca and Lawton were so open and willing to show us up close and personal how to prepare to die.

The insight we gained watching the way they loved each other was just remarkable. Their love was so strong you could feel it when you were with them. What a blessing from God that love was and is today for Jaca. Love like theirs doesn't end in death. It continues in the hearts and souls of those who are blessed enough to have lived it.

Balloons and a Birthday Cake

September 26, 2001

Lawton did not feel like having a party, but we couldn't let this important day go by without celebrating. We wanted Lawton to feel special. We bought an ice-cream cake and balloons and had a small party with a few friends. To see Lawton smile was the best part of the party.

Out to Dinner—only weeks before he died ...

Lawton could hardly walk, but he wanted to go out for dinner, and he wanted catfish. Catfish Country Restaurant was ten minutes away, so Jeff, Jaca, Lawton, Mary Jane, and I decided to have catfish for dinner. We always managed to find things to laugh about. We had a good time that night, and it was so good to see Jaca and Lawton laugh.

Special times like this are the memories I cherish.

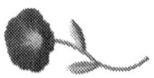

Mary Etta Darden—Reflections on Lawton DePriest

I remember the first sign of Lawton's sickness was the weight loss. When I asked him how he was losing so much weight (thinking he was dieting), in his usual quiet, slight smile, he just looked at Jaca and didn't say much. At that time I knew he was somewhat concerned, and it was the beginning of his many doctor appointments.

We watched over the next few months, and he was always upbeat and never seemed discouraged to our eyes.

I was in the hospital room the day the doctor came in and gave Jaca and Lawton the news he had a fatal disease. I must say I remember well the compassion of the doctor and the tears in his eyes. I never witnessed a doctor with that much feeling for his patient. I believe it was one thing that put Lawton at ease that day.

Lawton and Jaca were both amazingly calm after being told Lawton needed to go home and get his affairs in order. There were no tears or outburst—just a peace that only comes from a relationship with the Lord. I know they were in shock and didn't seem to hear everything the doctor was saying. When the doctor left, I also excused myself so they could have a few moments alone to digest what had been said. When I came back in the room they were both smiling and ready to face whatever was coming their way.

Within just a few minutes Lawton received a phone call from a golfing buddy, and I remember hearing for the first and only time any real displeasure at what was happening to him.

On later visits with Lawton at home, he was still upbeat and believing he could fight the battle. He was truly a witness to his faith in the Lord, and we will always remember him in the fondest way.

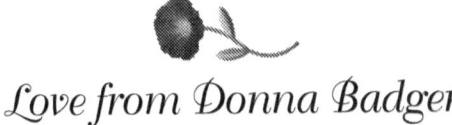

Love from Donna Badger

Since I did not have much time to sit down and quietly share my heart with you last night, the Lord woke me up very early this morning to do so. Our Lord placed on your heart the desire to write this precious book, and through the pages I have grown to love a man I never had the privilege to meet.

Having been through an adventure with cancer, this was a perfect picture of how I would have wanted to spend my last days on earth with Ted, had I known there were only a few remaining. It blessed my heart to read of your rock-solid commitment and love for both God and each other. It was inspiring to hear the specific and carefully thought-out plans you made together for your peace of mind. I believe God will use this blessing to strengthen and comfort couples who find themselves on the same journey, and it will also be a guidebook to the "beyond" that the Lord has planned for them. We, as readers, hear your heartfelt tears, prayers, and strong faith in the Lord. It will surely carry you through until the two of you meet again.

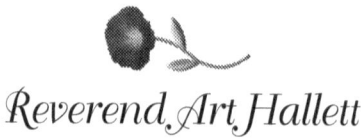

Reverend Art Hallett

Dear Jaca,

It was so good talking to you the other day. I'm just getting back to the office since we last talked. I've been traveling around the country and have been so very busy, but now I thought I'd take this moment to give you my note for your book on Lawton. Well, here goes.

The first time I met Lawton DePriest was after an invitation to stay with him and Jaca at their home in North Carolina. Lawton and Jaca knew of me through my music ministry at Bell Shoals Baptist Church in Brandon, Florida.

By an act of God Jill and I were invited to minister at Butner Federal Prison in Butner, North Carolina. It just so happened Lawton and Jaca now lived thirty minutes away from the prison. I thought that was great. So Lawton and Jaca invited us to stay in their home and volunteered to go to the prison with us to minister. Little did we know this was the beginning of a long-term relationship. We continued to visit the prison several times throughout the year, and Lawton and Jaca became regular volunteers with us.

At the prison Lawton was always so peaceful and merciful. I noticed immediately how he engaged the prisoners and demonstrated his ministry of mercy. He prayed and counseled with them every time we visited. The very first message I preached in the prison had a tremendous response from the inmates. Lawton also felt led of God to respond. I believe it was then Lawton came forward to confirm his faith in Christ. From that point on everything about him was amplified. His passion and love for the incarcerated or lost became more evident. I realize now that moment in prison had a tremendous impact on his life. And his life touched many others, some still incarcerated, but all have benefited from Lawton's ministry. It was such a joy to be around Lawton DePriest.

I really miss Lawton. Just writing this little note of praise to God makes me feel very blessed to have known Lawton and to have ministered alongside him. I look forward to a precious reunion with him one day in heaven.

God bless,
Art
Rev. Art Hallett
Sarasota, FL

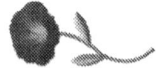

Lynn Mitchell—When to Say Good-bye

When a relative or close friend's death is imminent, when is the "right" time to say good-bye? How I would handle this issue weighed heavily on my mind.

Before a close relative (both my stepmother Major and then Lawton) was diagnosed with cancer, I had not witnessed the suffering and unending pain that often results. My Uncle Lawton gracefully accepted his prognosis and endured a painful ordeal lasting six long months. He was blessed with a loving wife of thirty plus years, and together they rode out the limited highs and the numerous lows. What I saw and felt each time I entered their home was an open, safe environment where visitors were always welcome. Lawton made a genuine effort to be an active participant in discussion regardless of the topic. If the discussion led to his health, that was all right. He kept no secrets. It was not difficult to keep conversations light, because their home was always warm and comfortable even though the suffering and changes of Lawton's physical being were painfully evident.

I frequently drew from Lawton's boundless wealth of knowledge concerning everything from where to buy a house after relocating to Brandon to an awesome recipe for turkey leftovers. I knew I could always count on him for well-thought-out advice or helpful suggestions. I needed to thank Lawton and let him know my appreciation for unselfishly sharing his infinite wisdom. But I wrestled with the timing. I decided to ask the advice of his wife and my mother as to when I should say good-bye. Their answer was sensible, but it did not make the approach any easier. However, the ever-present warm and welcoming atmosphere in their home was something I could always count on. The mood was never gloomy, because Lawton accepted his inevitable death with dignity, good spirits, and courage. His manner of facing death with both grace and acceptance was simply phenomenal. He was truly blessed with a caring, comforting physician, steadfast family members with him until the end, and a faithful loving wife who unselfishly provided gentle and vigilant care. As many dear friends dropped by to visit, warmth exuded from both Lawton and Jaca.

Lawton was truly genuine, and he always said what was on his mind. I made an effort to model myself after the example he set. His unshakeable genuineness is something that will always stick with me. I wondered why a kind and unselfish man would be taken from this earth at such an early age. It did not seem his unselfish giving and the assistance he provided should come to a close. He always had valuable information to share, and it was there for the asking. Though unfair as the situation seemed to me, the dismal circumstances of his condition were explained by his doctor and accepted by Lawton in an almost heroic way.

Being connected to a twenty-four hour intravenous line and in a constant nauseous state was surely an extraordinarily uncomfortable way to spend the last several months of life. But Lawton handled each stage with grace and dignity and no complaints. I truly felt the spiritual and psychological succor from following a terminally ill loved one through the last stages of life. Through this six month long process I somehow felt strengthened. When Jaca called to tell me of Lawton's passing, I was naturally overcome with great sadness. But partially traveling down the lonely road of losing this special loved one eased the initial pain. It seemed the grieving process began long before his death, and although his passing was heartbreaking, with it came a sense of peace and serenity.

Letting go is the difficult part of the journey, but when I witnessed gentleness and peace emanating from Lawton in his final days, I knew he was headed to a far greater place where eternal peace would finally be his.

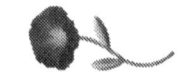

My Patient–Lawton DePriest

I am a surgical oncologist with a special interest in pancreatic cancer. Laypeople, or at least the "uninitiated" might describe my job as depressing or hopeless. Unfortunately for most of my patients, this perception is at least partly true. Lawton DePriest was one such patient who presented to me with advanced pancreatic cancer and a seemingly hopeless prognosis. After reading Jaca's account of Lawton's last days on this earth, I was not surprised to learn Lawton met the end of his life in much the same way he lived it.

I met Lawton in the emergency department of Tampa General Hospital. Just after completing nine years of training, I was eager to begin taking care of those patients whom I chose to spend the rest of my professional career caring for—patients with pancreatic cancer. My partner, Dr. Alexander Rosemurgy, is a nationally known surgeon due in part to his observations and skillful caring for these patients. He gave me some advice early on, and I specifically remember applying that advice to the care of Lawton DePriest. "Treat every patient as if they are your most important patient." When applying this philosophy to Lawton, I did not anticipate Lawton would teach me things about pancreatic cancer I could never learn in a textbook.

It became apparent early on Lawton would die of pancreatic cancer. His disease was advanced and inoperable. In the beginning he and Jaca desperately sought options that would provide hope despite his grim prognosis. But soon they accepted Lawton's terminal diagnosis. I saw Lawton frequently over the ensuing six months. I operated on him once. This was to bypass his stomach which was blocked by the growing cancer. He did well, and the operation provided him with some relief. Most importantly it allowed Lawton the ability to commune with his loved ones, share food, and fellowship. I believe this is a critical aspect of what validates and makes us human. It is something I try to prolong or maintain as long as possible in such patients.

Lawton's acceptance and approach to his illness was noteworthy. At first I thought he was simply putting his best foot forward when he visited in the clinic. He always looked well, had a smile on his face, and portrayed a good attitude. With each passing visit, I noted how his pants no longer fit, and how he was running out of holes on a belt that previously fit so snugly. When this happened, rather than drilling more holes into his belt as many patients do, Jaca took him out and bought him a new set of clothing. Many patients will dress in their finest clothing, they will wear cologne or perfume as foreign to them as their illness, and as a physician this behavior is extremely humbling. It is almost as if a patient is going to church. I realized Lawton was not disguising his true condition when he began to arrive more disheveled but with just as bright an attitude. As his disease began getting the better of him I saw he began to lose his verve, and I surmised the end was near.

In reading Jaca's account of Lawton's final days, his death was much as I imagined it would be—peaceful and accepting. Because Lawton accepted his diagnosis early, he had six months to prepare himself and Jaca for his terminal absence, and he did so with grace. As a result, Lawton died with a level of dignity difficult to find with this rapidly progressing disease. Most patients don't get beyond the anger phase before the disease catches up to them. When Lawton was told he wouldn't beat this diagnosis, he accepted the diagnosis, got to the business at hand, and accomplished most of what he set out to do.

People of faith will almost instinctively place themselves into the minority of patients who are expected to survive this diagnosis (which usually occurs through misdiagnosis). God-fearing people accept the diagnosis and move on. Lawton fell into the latter category. He never expected God to rescue him from his desperate situation. Lawton accepted his diagnosis as God's Divine providence, and he lived his remaining days in a manner suitable and worthy of God's will. This was very evident and very admirable. I won't ever forget Lawton. He was a critical early patient that influenced the way I have cared for each subsequent patient. Lawton could have written a textbook on living with a terminal diagnosis, as he did it with an instinct that was not contrived. I know in the end he was satisfied with his life on earth, and he was ready to enter into God's kingdom on his own terms. I will forever be indebted to Lawton for teaching me these valuable lessons about death, and more importantly, life.

—Emmanuel E. Zervos, MD, FACS
Professor of Surgery
Director, Division of Surgical Oncology
East Carolina University, Brody School of Medicine

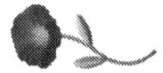

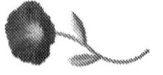

Reflections in the Beyond Days

The Quiet Times Alone

We shared everything in life. In death we can't share the glory, beauty, peace, and joy of heaven until we are both there. My heart aches for the moment we can once again be together and sharing life in our new home.

With each prayer came release of my Lawton.

You can virtually *feel* the Lord's feathers as His wings cover you, and He becomes your strong tower. Run to Him.

The thing with being a widow is you feel like no one needs you. It is almost impossible to find your place. More than half of you is gone. Now you are the only one remembering the memories, the sweet times, and all of the special things between you and your spouse that only the two of you shared.

Think of the language between two people whose lives are so inter-meshed. It is the language only the Lord can give. The prayers my Lawton and I shared were just such a language. We truly prayed exactly what was on our hearts. Our prayers were for each other and others, not for ourselves.

It took me so long to get to the place I knew my Lawton was facing imminent death. That's when the heart language really bloomed and blessed. It was the language that bound us closer together in the Lord and through which we were blessed.

If your loved one is approaching the end of life, please don't deny him or her the opportunity to grieve *with* you. Give them permission to talk about their illness, their emotions, their desire to see needs of their loved ones will be met after their death. These conversations will help you through the lonely days ahead. It is the legacy, the blessing, and the sharing of the most important time in your lives together. Please spend that time with them. Do not run from death, but instead, approach the time when Jesus comes to take your loved one by the hand.

What a release it was when I realized how important this phase is. Our Hospice nurse cried with me when I told her of Lawton and my prayer. His was for a pain-free, quick and soon home-going, and mine was to be by his side, telling him I loved him, and kissing his forehead. When I unwrap that gift the Lord gave to us, yes, many times there are tears. But that's not a bad thing at all. Tears heal, cleanse, and comfort.

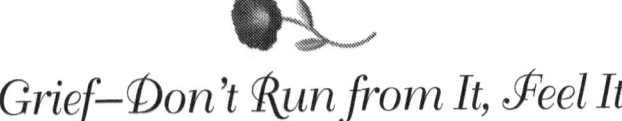

Grief—Don't Run from It, Feel It

Grief is very physical. It's not just emotional. Throughout Lawton's illness I was totally focused on his comfort and neglected my physical well-being. After his death, a dear friend kept telling me I should get a therapeutic massage. I'd never had one in my life, although I remember Lawton saying how beneficial it could be. Even his doctors prescribed back massages in the beginning of his illness. In my mind it didn't seem right having someone else (a perfect stranger) rub your back, neck, and arms.

At long last I decided it might help with my tired and aching body. The appointment was made with a highly recommended professional massage therapist. She is an RN and licensed massage therapist. We determined a deep tissue massage would be best considering the season of my life at the moment. It was immediately evident I had internalized deep emotions. I had tension you don't even recognize as tension. Gradually your shoulders slump and begin turning in and forward. It's as if your shoulders bend and try to cover your broken heart—as if protecting your most vulnerable spot.

For the next three months I went as often as I could afford it—almost every week. I went frequently in the following year, again as finances allowed. The good news is now some insurance companies cover this type of therapy if prescribed by your physician. Don't overlook this as not only a therapeutic healing but also an emotional step in dealing with your grief. Ask your doctor. It's infinitely better than anti-depressant medication.

We will all travel through our season of grief differently. This was something that was helpful to me and to many others. There is nothing in the rule book of grief to say you can or cannot do this or that or even keep the same traditions on holidays or other special days after the death of a loved one. You have the choice to begin new traditions if you want. Be creative. The most important thing to remember is to have a plan in place long before a special day arrives. You may not feel like following through with the plan, but do it anyway. It *will* make a difference.

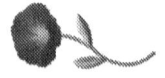

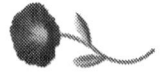

His Mercies Are New Every Day

Things People Did

- I received a personal care kit for the hospital that included tissues, lipstick, nail polish, emery board, lotion, small bud vase with a rosebud.

- Often I would return home to find balloons tied to the mailbox, flowers or a new plant by the front door.

- Hair cuts at home—our favorite hair stylist would often come by with scissors in hand offering a haircut.

- All kinds of meals—breakfast, lunch, dinner, and yummy desserts … lots of chocolate! Our freezer was stocked at all times.

- Lawn care—I'd hear a lawnmower and look out the window to see where it was. Lo and behold, it was my yard being mowed. Someone arranged for a lawn service during Lawton's illness.

- Notes—everyday there was a note in the mailbox. I still have them today.

- Phone calls—folks would visit via phone from all over the country.

- Visits—we loved having friends and family drop in. Usually they called first to make certain it was a good time. People made sure the visits were brief, no more than an hour unless asked to stay longer.

- Someone stayed with Lawton while I went to get my nails done or made a quick trip to the grocery.

- Give books of encouragement—often I read to Lawton. Sometimes he fell asleep while I read. Sometimes he had me repeat a paragraph as he pondered the words. Sometimes he just smiled and watched me read.

- Offer to take pets to the groomer or vet. We didn't have to worry when we were in the hospital, someone was always there to feed and let the dog out.

- If your church has video/DVD available of the Sunday worship service, make sure to provide a copy. Our church has a "Homebound Ministry." Lawton and I looked forward to the Sunday afternoon delivery of the video of the morning service.

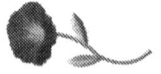

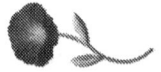

Enlarged Territory
... in the Beyond Days

A friend who is a "mobilizer" for those interested in short-term mission journeys mentioned an upcoming vision journey to the Middle East ministering to Muslim widows. Instantly my heart was touched and my interest was evident. She told me to pray, and we would talk in a couple of weeks.

Days later her husband mentioned he was blessed by my reaction to the trip. He told me more about the widows in the focus country. Again my heart jumped at the opportunity to reach out to these widows with the hope that lies within Christ Jesus. They are enveloped in such darkness because God's word is forbidden in their culture.

As time passed the trip proved extremely fluid as definite plans were not forthcoming. Although details of the journey were incomplete, it was certain that only a few would be able to go. Several ladies in our fellowship planned to go, and they encouraged me as I continued to seek God's will for my participation.

I am one of three women the Lord called to travel halfway across the world. The other two women were not the ones who originally committed to go. It is evident God called me to a group that has no age or geographic or ethnic boundaries—widows. The blessings continue, and I eagerly await the words and experiences He has for me as I build relationships with widows in this distant culture.

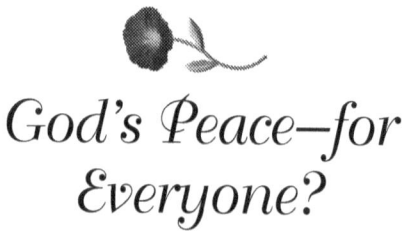

God's Peace—for Everyone?

Do you have the peace I've been writing about? Is there emptiness in your heart today? Do you have the assurance you will go to heaven when you die? May I share with you how to have peace that passes all understanding, how to fill the emptiness in your heart, and give you the blessed assurance you will spend eternity in heaven with the Lord Jesus?

God loves you and has a plan for your life. He created you for a purpose. This purpose was to have a personal relationship with Him.

Because of sin in your life, you are separated from God. We are all sinners. Romans 6:23 tells us,

> "The price of sin is death which is eternal separation from God." (Romans 6:23)

Even though sin separates man from God, there is hope. The price is already paid through Christ Jesus who loved you enough to die on the cross for your sins.

Eternal life is a free gift. You don't receive it by doing good things or trying to earn your way to heaven. There is only one way, and that's through Jesus. John 14:6 says, "I am the way, the truth, and the life. No one comes to the Father except through Me."

You must decide if you are willing to turn from your sins and ask Jesus into your heart with a simple prayer. "Jesus, I ask you into my heart to be my Savior and Lord. Forgive my sins, and give me the gift of eternal life."

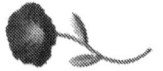

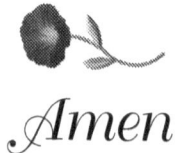

Amen

The beyond days continue. Even though my Lawton is no longer by my side, the Lord is forever with me. His Word says He will never leave or forsake me. I remember a quiet moment with the Lord about a year and a half after my Lawton died. My words were, "Father, Lawton and I shared everything in life. He is now having an experience I can't share. That makes me sad." In His gentle way the Lord reminded me I was having an experience Lawton could not share. He confirmed in my heart he was forever with me. Through the Lord we would always be together.

I find great comfort in knowing God still has me firmly in His grip. He is all I need. He faithfully supplies all our needs, and He genuinely wants to give us the desire of our hearts. Some days I don't know what I desire. Some days, He tells me my heart's desire. I look forward with great expectation and anticipation for the next revelation *Ah-Ha* moment as the Lord blesses me in these beyond days. I put one foot in front of the other and walk one step at a time. I was so blessed by God, my Lawton, family, friends, and other widows. I now live in the beyond days, secure in the knowledge I can go on.

> And not only this, but we also exult in our tribulations, knowing
> that tribulation brings about perseverance;
> and perseverance, proven character, and proven character, hope

and hope does not disappoint, because the love of God has been poured out within our hearts through the Holy Spirit who was given to us. (Rom. 5:3–5)

Be blessed in Him today. He loves you so!

Lawton and I shared an ordinary life. Our story is no different than hundreds or thousands of others. It's God's story, His story of grace, mercy, and peace as I lived it and am living it in the beyond.

For such is God, our God forever and ever; He will guide us until death. (Ps. 48:14)

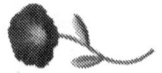

The days of October 2001 with family.

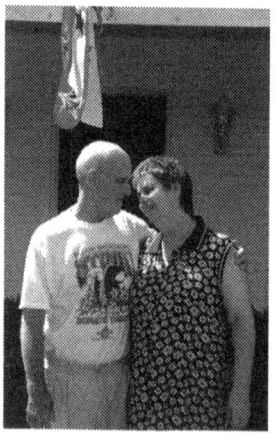

Lawton and Jaca

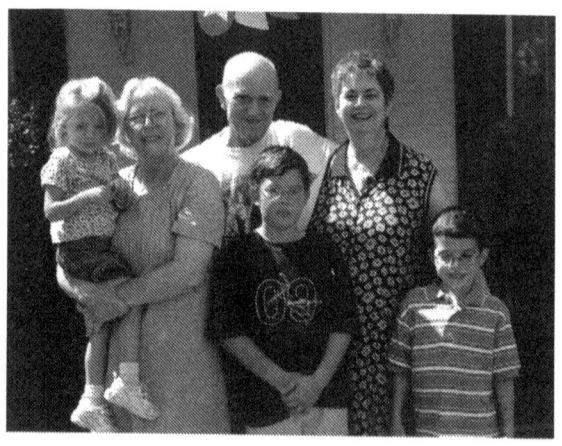

Kendall, Mary Jane, Nicholas, Jennings, Lawton, and Jaca

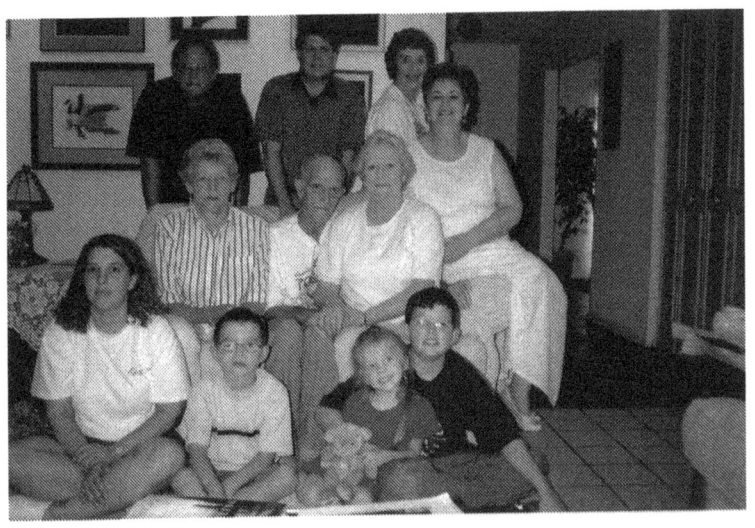

The family:
Fran, Jennings, Kendall, Nicholas, Aunt Ruby, Lawton, Mary Jane,
Jaca, Bob, Lawty, and Major

Before and After

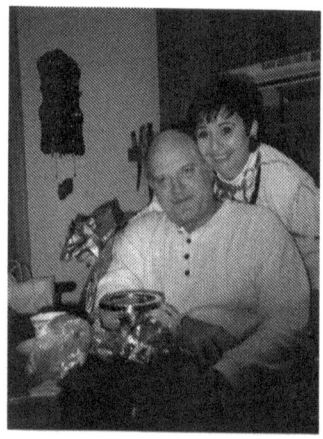

Lawton and Jaca—Christmas 1998

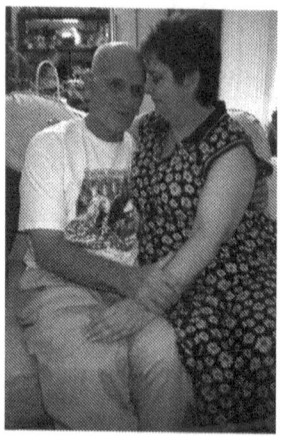

My Lawton and me as we begin the journey.

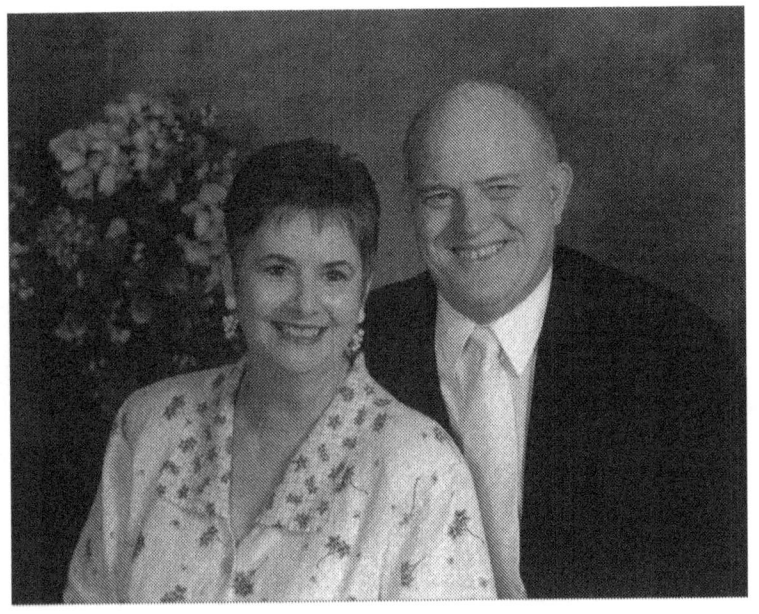

Lawton and Jaca—2000

978-0-595-41096-5
0-595-41096-0